Adriano Filipe Barreto Grangeiro

Functionality of the Elderly at Home in a Situation of Frailty

Adriano Filipe Barreto Grangeiro

Functionality of the Elderly at Home in a Situation of Frailty

Functional Capacity of the Elderly in Home Physiotherapy Programs in the Public and Private Sectors in Northeast Brazil

ScienciaScripts

Cover image: www.ingimage.com

This book is a translation from the original published under ISBN 978-3-330-75507-9.

Publisher:
Sciencia Scripts
is a trademark of
Dodo Books Indian Ocean Ltd. and OmniScriptum S.R.L publishing group

120 High Road, East Finchley, London, N2 9ED, United Kingdom
Str. Armeneasca 28/1, office 1, Chisinau MD-2012, Republic of Moldova, Europe
Printed at: see last page
ISBN: 978-620-8-26955-5

SUMMARY

I dedicate it to my dear and admirable maternal grandmother Vitorina Pereira Barreto (*In memorian*) who, during her 93 years, 7 months and 13 days here on earth, was an example of a warrior woman, brave, a fighter and kind to others. Thank you for your shared experience! I love you!

To my parents: Elcana Pereira Barreto Grangeiro and José Anilson Grangeiro, for the values and life lessons passed on to me throughout my life! Thank you for your constant presence in my education, always encouraging me, believing in me and helping to make my dreams come true!

To Emanuel Nogueira de Souza for accompanying me and always giving me his constant support! Your friendship, your example of optimism and faith, your dedication and your companionship have enabled me to get this far! Thank you for your patience, understanding and affection in times of distress! Eternally grateful to you!

To my siblings Anielle, Laudicéia, Jediel, Jeaias, Jesaias who have always supported me! Thank you for your love and friendship!

To my family, whom I love so much, my eternal dedication!

THANKS

To GOD, for remaining present in my life, guiding and illuminating my steps every day. Your love lasts forever! Thank you for loving me!

To Prof. Dr. Mônica Elinor Alves Gama, not just an advisor, but an excellent teacher, who accompanied me with her great wisdom, which was very useful to me, making herself present in my history and forever in my memory! Thank you for your dedication! Thank you for everything!

To the teachers of the Master's Degree Program in Adult and Child Health, who were responsible for the continuous learning, support, collaboration and teachings passed on along the way.

To my colleagues in class 10 of the Master's Program in Adult and Child Health for their friendship, strength and encouragement.

To my friends for their understanding!

To the Brazilian Society of Geriatrics and Gerontology - MA chapter for the encouragement to climb another step of knowledge!

To the General Director Fabiola Medeiros and the Administrative Director Genaina Moreira of the Center for Comprehensive Care of Elderly Health for opening the doors of the Center and giving us the kick-off of the research! Thank you for everything!

To the General Director of the Case Management Program of the Social Security Foundation - GEAP Cristiane for the space to start the research!

To the elderly interviewees and family members who allowed me to enter their homes, dedicating their time to answering the questionnaires and willingness to take part in this research! I was able to learn a lot from you, so you were fundamental to the conclusion of the data collection! Thank you for the information, affection, attention and support!

To everyone who contributed directly or indirectly, thank you very much!

"The art of growing old is the most delicate, the most subtle, the most indispensable if we are to be able to bring the journey of our time on earth to an end without disgrace."

(Alceu Amoroso Lima)

SUMMARY

Introduction: The growth of the elderly population is a worldwide phenomenon and one of the greatest challenges for public health, especially in developing countries such as Brazil. Significant changes in morbidity and mortality in this country are noticeable and can affect functionality, leading to a loss of autonomy and independence. Thus, evaluation studies that provide information on the specific characteristics of the elderly in terms of their ability to perform Basic Activities of Daily Living are fundamental for structuring prevention programs and making therapeutic decisions. **Objective: To** study the clinical and functional profile of frail elderly people treated at home in the public and private sectors in São Luis, MA. **Methods: This was** an analytical cross-sectional study. The sample consisted of 241 elderly people belonging to home physiotherapy programs in the public and private sectors. The data collection instruments used were: the Elderly Person's Health Booklet and the Barthel index. The data was analyzed using SPSS software. **Results:** Most of the elderly were women, aged 80-89, brown, retired, living with their families and requiring daily care. A significant association was found with the type of care provided in the public or private sector for the variables marital status (p=0.000), schooling (p=0.000) and monthly income (p=0.000). The main morbidities reported by the elderly in both groups were diseases of the circulatory system, with an average of 85.7% of those interviewed. There was a higher prevalence of elderly people in the private sector (57%) with total dependence to carry out Basic Activities of Daily Living and only 36.9% in the elderly in the public sector. In the elderly in the public sector there was a significant association with the occurrence of falls (p=0.0391), consumption of medication (p=0.0192) and previous hospitalization (p=0.0008) and in the elderly in the private sector the variables with a statistically significant difference were: occurrence of falls (p=0.0391) and consumption of medication (p=0.0192) when associated with degrees of functional dependence. **Conclusion:** A greater degree of dependence was found among the elderly in the private sector compared to the elderly in the public sector. This demonstrates the importance of prolonging and improving the quality of life of the elderly by expanding home-based programs with interdisciplinary assistance for this age group.

Keywords: Elderly health. Functional capacity. Physiotherapy. Quality of life.

1 INTRODUCTION

The Brazilian population has been aging rapidly and progressively. This is due to the fall in birth rates and the increase in life expectancy, progressively narrowing the base of the population pyramid (ARAUJO et al., 2011; STIVALI, 2011).

The process of population ageing is based on major political and socio-economic transformations that have led to changes in the demographic and epidemiological profiles of different societies, especially since the last century (FREESE AND FONTBONNE, 2006).

The World Health Organization (WHO) defines the elderly population as those aged 60 and over, but makes a distinction as to where the elderly reside. This limit is valid for developing countries and rises to 65 years of age in developed countries (WHO, 2009).

In Brazil, according to estimates projected for 2020, the number of elderly people over 60 years of age will be 28.3 million and, by 2050, approximately 64 million (FHON et al., 2012).

Age demographic data shows that the elderly are the fastest growing part of the population worldwide. Data from the Brazilian Institute of Geography and Statistics (IBGE) show that the widening of the top of the age pyramid can be seen in the growth in the relative share of the population aged 65 and over, which was 4. 8% in 1991, rising to 5.9% in 2000 and reaching 7.4% in 2007,8% in 1991, rising to 5.9% in 2000 and reaching 7.4% in 2010, and the Southeast and South are the oldest Brazilian regions, where 8.1% of the population is made up of elderly people aged 65 or over (IBGE, 2010).

According to the National Household Sample Survey (PNAD) carried out in 2013, the number of people aged 60 or over rose from 9.0% to 13% of the total population between 2001 and 2013.

Brazil is rapidly moving towards a more aged demographic profile, characterized by an epidemiological transition in which Chronic Degenerative Diseases, also known as Chronic Non-Communicable Diseases (CNCD), occupy a prominent place. The increase in chronic diseases means that public policies need to be adapted, particularly those aimed at meeting the growing demands in the areas of health, welfare and social assistance (MENDES, 2011).

According to data from the 2010 Census, the population of elderly people in the state of Maranhão represents 568,681 (8.3%), with the city of São Luis comprising 77,971 elderly people, i.e. a percentage of 7.4% (IBGE, 2013).

In the area of health, this rapid demographic and epidemiological transition poses major challenges, as it is responsible for the emergence of new health demands, especially the "Epidemic of Chronic Diseases and Functional Disabilities", resulting in greater and longer use of health services (MORAES, 2012).

NCDs can affect the functionality of older people. Studies show that dependence for the performance of Activities of Daily Living (ADLs) tends to increase from around 5% in the 60s to around 50% among those aged 90 or over (BRASIL, 2010).

As we get older, the prevalence of chronic diseases in the elderly increases. Studies have shown that more than 70% of the elderly have some kind of illness. The greater the number of chronic diseases affecting the elderly, the greater the prevalence of impairments that can lead to functional incapacity (BARROS et al., 2006; ALVES et al., 2007; TRIBESS et al., 2009).

Loss of functional capacity is associated with a predisposition to frailty, dependence, institutionalization, increased risk of falls, death and mobility problems, bringing complications over time and generating long-term care and high costs (MACIEL E GUERRA, 2007).

The ageing process brings about changes which, together with the increase in the prevalence of chronic non-communicable diseases, can lead to the appearance of Geriatric Syndromes, among which the Frailty Syndrome stands out (VERAS, 2009).

According to Freitas et al. (2006), the elderly have various health needs, especially the frail elderly, who are extremely vulnerable to a deterioration in their functional capacity.

The National Health Policy for the Elderly (PNSPI), Ordinance GM No. 2.528, of October 19, 2006, considers frail elderly people to be those who: lives in Long Stay Institutions for the Elderly (ILPI), is bedridden, has recently been hospitalized for any reason, has diseases known to cause functional incapacity such as (Encephalic Vascular Accident, Dementia Syndromes and other Neurodegenerative Diseases, Alcoholism, Terminal Neoplasia, Limb Amputations), has at least one basic functional incapacity, or experiences domestic violence. By age criterion, the literature establishes that the elderly aged 75 or over are also frail. Other criteria can be added or modified according to local realities (MINISTÉRIO DA SAÙDE, 2006).

According to Brasil (2010), the Caderneta de Saùde da Pessoa Idosa (Elderly Person's Health Booklet) is considered a valuable tool to help identify elderly people who are frail or at risk of frailty. This instrument was developed by the Ministry of Health in 2007 with the aim of assessing items relating to the functional capacity of the elderly.

Another instrument developed to assess functional capacity is the Barthel index (BI), used in this study. According to Minosso et al. (2010), the BI belongs to the field of ADL assessment and measures the degree of assistance required by an individual in personal care, mobility, locomotion and elimination. Functional independence is assessed through 10 tasks: feeding, bathing, dressing, personal hygiene, bowel movements, bladder movements, toilet use, chair-bed passage, ambulation and stairs.

Assessing functional condition is essential when formulating policies for the health of the elderly. Studies aimed at contributing to improvements in policies for the health care of the elderly should take a close look at the functional aspect (FERNANDES, 2010).

Brazil, concerned about the impact of the population ageing process, created the National Policy for the Elderly (PNI) in 1994 with the aim of ensuring the social rights of the elderly, creating conditions to promote their autonomy, integration and effective participation in society, reaffirming their right to health at the various levels of care (SANTOS et al., 2008). Among the PNI's priorities is the stimulation of Home Care, valuing the favorable effect of the family environment on the recovery process of the elderly and providing benefits for them and for the Health System (SOUZA E CALDAS, 2008).

Ordinance No. 73 of May 10, 2001 (BRASIL, 2001) lays down the rules for the operation of Services for the Care of the Elderly in Brazil and defines Home Care as care provided to elderly people with some level of dependency, with the aim of increasing the autonomy of the elderly so that they can remain living in their homes for as long as possible.

Based on this ordinance, Home Care is characterized as:

> "A public or private home care service for the elderly through an individualized program, of a preventive and rehabilitative nature, in which a network of services and professional intervention techniques focused on health care, personal, domestic, psychosocial and family support, and interaction with the community are articulated. It can be of a permanent or temporary nature, daytime and/or nighttime, for dependent or semi-dependent elderly people, with or without resources and with or without family ties" (BRASIL, 2001, p.44).

Later, other programs, such as the National Health Policy for the Elderly, reinforced this home care (BRASIL, 2010). The Home Care Service at the Hospital do Servidor Pùblico municipal de Sâo Paulo began its activities in 1994, demonstrating the importance of home care as an alternative to the high cost of hospitalizations and the impact on the elderly population of the expenses resulting from these hospitalizations (LEME E DIAS, 2007).

Studies show that as the population ages, the proportion of elderly people with sequelae of Chronic-Degenerative Diseases progressively increases, which generally contributes to their dependence in carrying out Basic Activities of Daily Living, so every day Home Care deserves more emphasis with progressive expansion (BARCELOS E MADUREIRA, 2009).

Home physiotherapy programs have been growing in many countries, such as Brazil, and there are many reasons why patients or their families choose this type of care, from physical and functional incapacity, such as a bed restriction that prevents or hinders mobility, to the convenience and practicality of this type of care (SILVA et al., 2011).

Considering that increased longevity is associated with frailty and functional incapacity in the elderly, they are more exposed to risks, it is therefore important to carry out research on this topic, so that health actions can be planned and offer the frail elderly a place to live with better living conditions (FHON et al., 2012).

Thus, the experience of home care for the elderly in situations of frailty in home physiotherapy programs motivated the study of this topic due to the growth of the aging population, which leads to an increase in chronic non-communicable diseases, reducing the functional capacity of this age group, causing a loss of autonomy and independence.

Evaluative studies that provide insight into the specific characteristics of elderly people in situations of frailty in relation to their ability to perform the Basic Activities of Daily Living are fundamental for structuring prevention programs and making therapeutic decisions.

2 THEORETICAL BACKGROUND

2.1 Old age and aging

In order to gain a better understanding of the research carried out, it is necessary to know who the elderly are within the process of old age and ageing. This sub-item deals with the concepts of the elderly, old age and ageing, showing their classification.

The elderly are populations or individuals who can be characterized by the length of their life cycle. [...] Gender, social class, health, education, personality factors, past history and socio-historical context are important elements that combine with chronological age to determine differences between the elderly aged between 60 and 100 (NERI, 2001).

The WHO defines the elderly as anyone aged 65 or over living in developed countries and 60 or over living in developing countries (MAZO et al., 2001).

According to the Statute of the Elderly, published in 2003, the elderly are considered to be people aged 60 or over, of both sexes, without distinction of color, race or ideology.

From conception to death, the human organism goes through various stages: development, puberty, maturity and ageing (PAPALÉO NETTO, 2007).

Aging is a vital process inherent to all human beings. Old age is a stage of life, an integral part of a natural cycle, constituting a unique and differentiated experience (SILVA, 2009).

For the WHO, old age is: "[...] the prolongation and termination of a process represented by a set of physiomorphic and psychological modifications uninterrupted by the action of time on people" (ARAÙJO, 2001).

Old age is characterized by biological, psychological, cognitive and social changes that increase predisposition to situations of functional incapacity, multimorbidity and increased risk of vulnerability. These very diverse and individual changes make ageing a heterogeneous and subjective experience

(TEIXEIRA, 2007).

Beauvoir (1970, p.17) states that, "old age is not a static fact; it is the end and prolongation of a process, a process called ageing".

Ageing can be understood as:

> A natural process of progressive decline in the functional reserve of individuals called senescence which, under normal conditions, does not usually cause any problems. However, under conditions of overload, such as illness, accidents and emotional stress, it can lead to a pathological condition that requires assistance called senility (BRASIL, 2010, p.8).

The Pan American Health Organization (PAHO) defines ageing as a sequential, individual, accumulative, irreversible, non-pathological process of deterioration of a mature organism, typical of all members of a species, so that time makes it less able to cope with the stress of the environment and therefore increases the possibility of death (GONTIJO, 2005).

Ageing is interpreted as:

> A multidimensional process, it results from the interaction of biological, psycho-emotional and socio-cultural factors. The other factors are individual and social compositions, the result of visions and opportunities that each society attributes to its elderly (SALGADO, 2007, p.68).

According to Tammaro et al. (apud SANTANA, 2001) ageing can be classified into the following phases: *Middle age* - which covers the period between 45 and 60 years of age, also known as pre-senile *age*. During this phase, important biological events occur, such as the menopause for women and the andropause for men. *Gradual senescence* - between the ages of 65 and 75, a phase in which potential pathologies easily manifest themselves. *Senescence proper* - between 75 and 90 years of age. In this phase, the individual presents physiopathological changes, with a reduced functional reserve, associated with a fragile and unstable biological balance.

There is a consensus on aging patterns, understood from three aspects:

> a) As a universal and progressive phenomenon that presents a gradual decrease in the individual's ability to adapt, it is called *primary aging*; b) As a phenomenon with changes caused by diseases associated with aging, such as cancer and coronary heart disease, among others, it is called *secondary aging*; c) The so-called *tertiary* or terminal *aging* is a phenomenon where great physical and cognitive loss is noticed in a relatively

short period of time, usually leading to death (ROLIM E FORTI, 2004, p.58-59).

Mazo et al. (2001) report that these patterns and definitions are influenced by social, biological, intellectual and functional components and can therefore be recognized as biological ageing, social ageing, intellectual ageing and functional ageing.

In order to understand the ageing process, it is necessary to have an understanding of the totality and complexity of the human being, since each aspect, be it biological, cultural or social, is not disconnected. In this way, we understand the cycles that human beings go through during their existence (ARALDI, 2008).

2.2 Population Ageing

The growing number of elderly people around the world, proven by numerous demographic and epidemiological studies, has presented government bodies and society with the medical and socio-economic challenges of an ageing population (PAPALÉO NETTO, 2007).

Between the 1940s and 1970s, there was a huge increase in the population's life expectancy, due to Public Health actions such as vaccinations and basic sanitation, as well as technological advances (FONSECA, 2000).

In the 1970s, the growth of the elderly population was more significant in Europe, Japan and North America (NETTO, 2001).

In 1980, the population aged 65 and over represented 15.5% of the inhabitants of Federal Germany, 13.5% of the population of France and Italy, 11.4% of the United States, 8.2% of Argentina and 3% of African countries (GRIFFA, 2011). "[...] it can be inferred that ageing can no longer be considered the preserve of developed countries" (CARVALHO FILHO E PAPALÉO NETO, 2000).

The growth of the elderly population has shown a surprising acceleration, especially in developing countries (SANTANA et al., 2009), as is the case in Brazil.

In Brazil, as the percentage of elderly people increases, the proportion of younger people decreases. Two fundamental factors explain this type of fluctuation: the fall in fertility, responsible for the reduction in the percentage of the younger age group, and the fall in mortality, responsible for the increase in the percentage of the elderly (PAPALÉO NETO, 2007, p.9).

The changes that have been taking place in the population pyramid show that the number of people aged 65 or over has risen from 3% in 1991 and 3.6% in 2000 to 4.6% in 2010 (IBGE 2010).

The World Bank Report (IBRD, 2011) released in 2011 shows that Brazil is aging much faster than developed countries. According to the survey, rich nations first became rich, then old. Brazil and other emerging countries are getting old before they get rich. While it took France more than a century to increase from 7% to 14% of the population aged 65 and over, Brazil will go through the same process in two decades, from 2011 to 2031. Over the next 40 years, the Brazilian population as a whole will grow at an average of just 0.3% a year, while the elderly will grow at a rate of 3.2% - 10 times more. Thus, the elderly, who were 4.9% of the population in 1950 (and took 60 years to double that proportion), will triple to 29.7% by 2050.

The results of the 2010 Census show that Brazil has 190,755,799 inhabitants, of which 20,590,599 are considered elderly (aged ≥ 60) and that the Brazilian population has grown by 12.3% over the last decade, at an average rate of 1.17% per year. This population includes 13.8 million children under the age of four (3.6%) and 14 million people over the age of 65 (7.4%) (IBGE, 2010).

The Northeast region, which had the lowest life expectancy at birth in 1980 (58.25 years) had a 12.95 year increase in this indicator in 30 years, reaching 71.20 years in 2010, slightly above the North region, which was previously ahead of it (from 60.75 years to 70.76 years). This inversion was mainly due to the 14.14-year increase in life expectancy among women in the northeast, from 61.27 years to 75.41, while that of women in the North increased by 10.62 years, from 63.74 to 74.36 years (IBGE, 2013).

It is estimated that, by 2025, Brazil will rank sixth in terms of the number of elderly people, with around 32 million people aged 60 or over. In 2050, children aged 0 to 14 will represent 13.15%, while the elderly population will reach 22.71% of the total population (MORAES, 2012).

Considering the increase in the elderly population, both in developed and developing countries, it is important to be concerned about the speed at which the number of elderly people in Brazilian society is increasing and the consequences that this phenomenon entails (FREITAS et al., 2011).

The phenomenon of ageing is an undeniable reality, and projections indicate that this growth will continue apace, especially in developing countries such as Brazil (IBGE, 2010).

In this way, profound and immediate reformulations of social and health policies become necessary, so that we can absorb, at least in part, the impact of the galloping demographic transition and, only in this way, prevent the extra years of life gained from being synonymous with the accumulation of disabilities and dependencies, thus greatly compromising the quality of life of the majority of the elderly (PAPALÉO NETTO, 2007).

2.3 Physiological and Functional Aspects of Ageing

Physiological ageing comprises a series of alterations in organic functions due exclusively to the effects of advanced age on the body, causing it to lose its ability to maintain homeostatic balance and all physiological functions to gradually begin to decline (STRAUB, R. H., CUTOLO, M., ZIETZ, B et al. 2010).

> Organic functions generally decline over time. This decline, however, is quite variable when you consider the rate of deterioration in different organ systems and in different individuals. It is generally accepted that every year, from the age of 30, there is a loss of 1% of function (PAPALÉO NETO, 2007, p.6).

The decline in organic functions, systems and physiological reserves therefore makes the individual more predisposed to chronic conditions (MARQUES, 2001).

In the elderly, the main chronic health conditions are represented by diseases or comorbidities, disabilities, frequent symptoms, self-medication, iatrogeny and the very vulnerability associated with ageing (MORAES, 2012).

Chronic conditions and the natural aging process itself reduce the functional capacity of each of the body's systems, accentuating functional aging (GOMES, 2012).

Functionality is one of the fundamental attributes of human ageing, as it deals with the interaction between physical and psychocognitive abilities to carry out everyday activities and health conditions, an interaction mediated by the skills and competencies developed throughout the life course (PERRACINI et al., 2009, p.7).

In this way, the focus of health is strictly related to the individual's overall functionality, defined as the ability to manage one's own life or take care of oneself. A person is considered healthy when they are able to carry out functional activities independently and autonomously, even if they have illnesses. This has profound consequences for the structure of healthcare networks (MORAES, 2012).

Functional capacity is defined as the ability to maintain the necessary physical and mental activities, which means being able to live independently for Basic and Instrumental Activities of Daily Living. This impairment has implications for the elderly, their families, the community and the health system, since disability leads to greater dependence and vulnerability in old age (FHON et al., 2012).

The day-to-day tasks required for individuals to look after themselves and their own lives are called Activities of Daily Living (ADLs). They can be classified according to their degree of complexity into basic, instrumental and advanced. The greater the complexity of ADLs, the greater the need for the main functional systems (cognition, mood, mobility and communication) to function properly, in an integrated and harmonious way (MORAES, 2012, p.11-12).

With advancing age, around 10.0% of the population need help with Basic Activities of Daily Living (BADL), such as feeding, bathing, dressing, going to the toilet and getting around (KARSCH, 2003).

Fiedler and Peres (2008) identified in a group of elderly people that the age variable is strongly associated with loss of functionality, as the group aged 70 or over had a greater chance of impaired functionality when compared to those aged between 60 and 69.

One in nine elderly people between the ages of 65 and 74 had difficulty performing basic functional tasks and consider that mobility and movement are essential for carrying out these activities. Restrictions in the elderly can lead to dependency, reduced autonomy and social interaction, interfering with self-esteem and well-being (PEREIRA E GOMES, 2004).

Based on this, functional capacity has emerged as a new health paradigm, proposed by the National Health Policy for the Elderly (PNSPI). Independence and autonomy for as long as possible are goals to be achieved in Health Care for the Elderly (BRASIL, 2010).

2.4 Functional Capacity, Autonomy and Independence

The International Classification of Functioning (ICF) defines functional capacity as the ability to perform a task or action, aiming to indicate the probable maximum level of functionality that the individual can achieve in a given domain at a given time (KAWASAKI & DIOGO, 2004).

According to Freitas and Miranda (2011), "Functional capacity is defined as the ability of the elderly to perform a certain task that allows them to take care of themselves and lead an independent life".

The WHO has proposed a model to illustrate the slow and progressive decline in general functions that occurs in early adulthood, represented by figure 1, which shows the curve of functional capacity throughout the life course (PERRACINI et al., 2009).

Figure 1: Functional Capacity Curve over the life course.

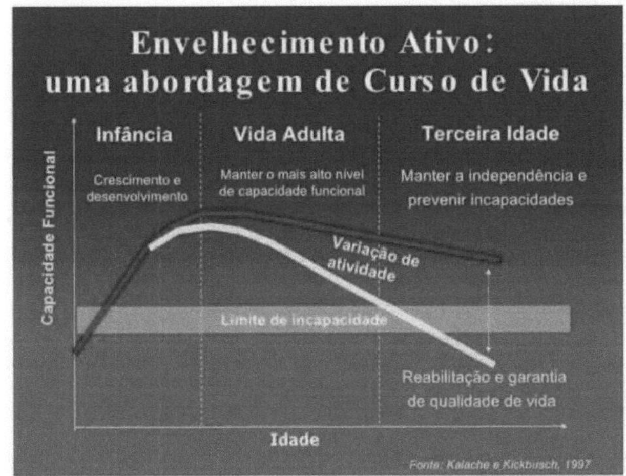

Source: Kalache and Kickbuschh. Active Ageing: a policy framework, 1997.

In old age, a healthier life is closely linked to maintaining or restoring autonomy and independence (PASCHOAL, 2005), which are defined as follows: autonomy is the individual's ability to make decisions and take control of actions, establishing and following their own rules, and independence is the ability to accomplish something with their own means, allowing the individual to take care of themselves and their life (MORAES, 2012).

It should be noted that functional capacity can be an important indicator of health and quality of life, as it considers aspects related to the independence and autonomy of the elderly person within their social environment (VERAS, 2002; MORAES, 2008) and in gerontology, assessing functionality is extremely important, as performance in ADLs has become a widely accepted and recognized reference, as it allows health professionals a more accurate view of the severity of the disease and its sequelae (RICCI, et al., 2005).

"Elderly people with numerous comorbidities, especially chronic diseases, may have difficulties in performing ADLs" (PARKER AND THORSLUND, 2007). Based on this assumption, it is necessary to have an idea of what kind of care or help the individual needs, and it is essential to assess their functionality, which is based on their ability to perform ADLs (MOTTA et al., 2013), which according to Carleto et al. (2010), are divided into:

- Basic Activities of Daily Living (BADLs) or Personal Activities of Daily Living (PADLs): these are activities that focus on the individual's care of their own body and are considered fundamental to life in the social world, as they allow for survival and well-being, being self-care tasks, such as eating, dressing up and down, functional mobility, care of personal equipment, personal hygiene, sphincter control, bathing and using the toilet;

- Instrumental Activities of Daily Living (IADL) or Practical Life Activities (PLA): these are activities that support daily life in the home and in the community, which often require more complex interactions than the self-care used in ADL. These include household chores, shopping, managing one's own medication, handling money, preparing one's own meals, tidying the house, washing and ironing;

- Advanced Activities of Daily Living refer to social integration. These activities are extremely individualized and difficult to generalize. Productive activities, social activities, recreational activities, formal and informal work, driving, voluntary service, organizing events, using technology (internet) and hobbies are examples of advanced activities of daily living. Hence the importance of knowing prior functionality, which is the only way to compare the individual with themselves and recognize the presence of functional decline (MORAES, 2012).

Using appropriate tools, it is possible to effectively determine the main losses in functional capacity, the order in which they appear, the intensity of these losses, the need to adapt to the environment and how the family can help to reduce these problems (TORRES, 2010).

The same author points out that maintaining the functional capacity of the elderly, according to the individuality and specificity of each situation, is one of the most important roles of family members, caregivers and health professionals, deserving a special focus on the multidisciplinary approach of this age group, aiming above all to provide a better quality of life in the face of loss of functional capacity.

2.5 Functional assessment of the elderly

The functional assessment recommended by the PNSPI is fundamental and will determine not only the functional impairment of the elderly person, but also their need for assistance. It can be understood as a systematized attempt to objectively assess the levels at which a person is functioning in a variety of areas using different skills. It represents a way of measuring whether or not a person is able to perform the activities necessary to look after themselves (BRASIL, 2010).

Ramos (2003) points to the importance of assessing functional capacity as a new paradigm for public health in the face of ageing, in which the concept of health is changing towards the maintenance of autonomy, regardless of the presence of controlled chronic diseases.

There are numerous instruments for assessing the functional status of the elderly and many are applied without a prior study of their psychometric measures. The appropriate choice of instrument certainly depends on the operating environment and the objectives of the study. However, the correct selection presupposes formal knowledge of the validity and reliability results of the instrument in question (LITVOC E BRITO, 2004).

The Barthel index was therefore chosen for this study, as it is a widely used instrument worldwide for assessing functional independence and mobility.

A review study on instruments for assessing the functional status of the elderly, carried out in 2004, identified this index as one of the most widely used instruments for assessing Activities of Daily Living (PAIXAO JUNIOR E REICHENHEIM, 2005).

The Barthel index measures the degree of assistance required by an individual in personal care, mobility, locomotion and elimination. Functional independence is assessed using 10 tasks: eating, bathing, dressing, personal hygiene, bowel movements, bladder movements, using the toilet, moving from chair to bed, walking and stairs (MINOSSO et al., 2010).

Each item of the instrument is scored according to the patient's performance in carrying out tasks independently, with some help or dependently (MC DOWEL AND NEWELL, 1996).

Other tools have been developed by the Ministry of Health (MS) to evaluate items relating to the functionality of the elderly, including the Caderneta de Saùde da Pessoa Idosa.

Launched in 2007 by the Ministry of Health to be adopted in all the country's Basic Health Units, the Caderneta de Saùde da Pessoa idosa (BRASIL, 2007) captures items about the socioeconomic characterization, life habits and health of the elderly.

The Caderneta de Saùde da Pessoa Idosa is a valuable tool that makes it possible to plan and organize actions and better monitor the state of health of this age group, representing an important instrument for strengthening primary care (BRASIL, 2010).

In 2012, the Ministry of Health made available the new Caderneta de Saùde da Pessoa Idosa (Elderly Person's Health Booklet) with items on day-to-day care, assessing the Basic and Instrumental Activities of Daily Living, observing whether the elderly person is capable of carrying out this activity, or whether they have any difficulties or are incapable. It also assesses memory and communication problems, oral health, the presence of risk situations for frailty and diagnoses the elderly person's risk of frailty (BRASIL, 2012).

In this way, we can consider functional assessment as one of the main elements of the clinical assessment of the elderly, and it is fundamental for making therapeutic decisions. Functional impairment has a significant negative impact on the quality of life of the elderly, impairing their daily lives and causing vulnerability and dependence. It also has negative repercussions for family members, the community and the health system (SANTOS E GAETA, p.8).

It is in this context that the so-called "functional assessment" becomes essential for establishing an appropriate diagnosis, prognosis and clinical judgment, which will serve as the basis for decisions on the treatment and care needed by the elderly. It is a parameter which, together with other health indicators, can be used to determine the effectiveness and efficiency of proposed interventions (BRASIL, 2010).

Verifying the loss of functional capacity in the elderly through a functional assessment with a multi-professional team allows for the construction of appropriate interventions as early as possible that will benefit the elderly, allowing them to maintain a satisfactory quality of life, with active ageing (TORRES, 2010).

3 OBJECTIVES

3.1 **General**

To study the clinical and functional profile of frail elderly people assisted in public and private sector home physiotherapy programs in the municipality of São Luis, Maranhão.

3.2 **Specifics**

- To describe the sociodemographic characteristics of the population studied;
- To identify health problems, the occurrence of previous hospitalizations and self-reported falls by the elderly;
- To identify the lifestyle habits and the practice of regular physical activity self-reported by the elderly;
- Assess the degree of functional dependence of the elderly person.

4 METHODOLOGY

4.1 Type of study

Analytical cross-sectional study.

4.2 Study period and location

This was a study carried out from April to September 2014 with elderly people assisted in the Home Care Program for the Frail Elderly (PADIF) and the Case Management Program (PGC) in Sâo Luis, Maranhâo.

PADIF is a type of home care in the public sector, developed by the Municipal Health Department of the municipality of Sâo Luis, Maranhâo, maintained with resources from the Unified Health System, operating in the Center for Comprehensive Care for the Health of the Elderly, which provides biopsychosocial and spiritual care to elderly people in situations of frailty, carried out by a multi-professional team made up of:

- 01 Doctor[1]
- 01 Nurse and
- 01 Physiotherapist[2]

Each patient is treated within 60 days, or two months.

PADIF has been in operation since February 2009 and the elderly are included in the program's actions by registering and filling out a specific form sent to the Center for Comprehensive Health Care for the Elderly, which requests a home visit.

Upon receiving the demand, it is identified whether it meets the criteria for inclusion in the program:

- Elderly (60 years or older) living in São Luis (02 points);

1 Geriatrician certified by the Brazilian Society of Geriatrics and Gerontology.
2 Specialist in Gerontology by the Brazilian Society of Geriatrics and Gerontology.

- Bedridden (04 points);
- Victim of violence (04 points);
- Area discovered by the Family Health Strategy (03 points).

If the elderly person's score is above six points, they will be referred to the PADIF team to be included in the home visit program, and a monthly schedule will be drawn up.

The PGC of a health plan is a private home care service aimed at individuals of any age who need special attention due to chronic, degenerative, serious or terminal illnesses, carried out by a multidisciplinary team, with the aim of promoting, maintaining or restoring health or minimizing the effects of illnesses and disabilities, with the participation of the family and/or caregiver. It is represented by a coordinator and two teams of professionals made up of:

- 04 Doctors[3]
- 02 Nurses[4]
- 02 Nursing Technicians
- 06 Physiotherapists[5]
- 05 Speech therapists
- 04 Occupational Therapists[6]
- 02 Psychologists[7]
- 02 nutritionists.

Each patient is seen up to four times a week, totaling a maximum of 15 and a minimum of 5 monthly rehabilitation treatment appointments. Doctors, nurses and nutritionists provide a monthly service.

---

3 03 specialists in clinical medicine and 01 specialist in Social Gerontology and Elderly Health.
4 01 specialist in Social Gerontology and Elderly Health.
5 03 specialists in Gerontology, 01 of whom has a degree from the Brazilian Society of Geriatrics
6 02 Gerontology specialists.
7 01 specialist in Gerontology.

The PGC has been running since July 2002. For the selection of cases, the team responsible for the program will consider the sum of the following criteria:

I. Clinical-epidemiological criteria - are a priority in the assessment scale. The beneficiary may have one of the following profiles, as long as their clinical condition is stable and they do not need equipment and/or technological resources for their care or a health team on call at home.

a. Beneficiaries with Chronic, Degenerative and Severe Diseases, with a high rate of use of Health Services or frequent readmissions, except psychiatric patients;

b. Beneficiaries with a disability who have suffered from an illness or the sequelae of an illness, have been treated, but have suffered a permanent disability, such as quadriplegics, paraplegics, stroke victims and amputees.

c. Beneficiaries who have had an illness or the sequelae of an illness or have undergone major surgery, have been treated and have acquired clinical stability but have suffered long-term complications, such as burns, orthopedic polytrauma, people with infections that require extensive debridement and drainage and stomas, and people with diabetic feet and/or varicose ulcers;

d. Terminally ill beneficiaries who are beyond therapeutic possibilities and require general care and symptom relief, such as neoplasms, chronic lung disease, chronic kidney disease and AIDS, provided that the beneficiary and/or their family agree to be de-hospitalized. e. Cases that are not included in the above situations will be studied individually and, according to the opinion of the Health Promotion Coordination, may or may not be included in the Program.

e. Cases that are not included in the above situations will be studied individually and, according to the opinion of the Health Promotion Coordination, may or may not be included in the Program.

II. Geographical criteria

a.Capital and metropolitan region, except in places that are difficult to access.

4.3 Study sample

The sampling method was systematic probabilistic, with those assessed being sorted alphabetically and then drawn by lot using a withdrawal interval of ***k=3***. Consequently, the final sample of 241 elderly people was obtained.

The inclusion criteria for the study were defined as: elderly people of both sexes, aged 60 or over, living in the area covered by the municipality of São Luis, registered and followed up in Home Physiotherapy Programs for a period of six months or more.

Elderly people who did not meet these criteria were excluded from the study.

4.4 Sample size calculation

Considering the monthly visits to home care services in the public sector (n=32) and the private sector (n=71) over a six-month period of data collection between April and September 2014, a total of approximately 618 elderly people were seen in the two programs over this period.

With a sampling error of 5%, a statistical power of 95%, and finally a prevalence of 37% of some degree of dependence using the Barthel index described by Minosso et al. (2010), a sample of 241 elderly people was estimated.

4.5 Instruments used for data collection

The first instrument used for data collection was the Caderneta de Saùde da Pessoa Idosa (Elderly Person's Health Booklet) (ANNEX A), made available by the Ministry of Health as part of a strategy for monitoring the health of the population, covering sociodemographic data and using the 37

the following variables: gender, age, color, marital status, schooling, occupational status, monthly income, number of people living in the household, personal morbidity data, lifestyle habits such as smoking, drinking and physical activity, occurrence of falls, health problems according to the International Statistical Classification of Diseases and Related Health Problems - Tenth Revision (ICD-10), use of medication and hospital admissions.

The Barthel index (ANNEX B) was used to assess the degree of functional dependence and comprises a 10-item assessment of ADLs involving mobility and personal care (O'SULLIVAN et al, 2004).

The elderly person's health booklet was filled in at the time of the home visit. If the elderly person at home was unable to communicate or had difficulties, a caregiver or guardian answered the questions. The interviews were carried out by interviewers who were university-educated health professionals. They were trained to apply the booklet and were assessed and monitored throughout the research period.

The WHO definition for developing countries was used, which considers elderly people to be those aged 60 or over.

The health problem variable included signs, symptoms, diseases diagnosed or self-reported by the elderly or their guardians.

The analysis of risk factors contained in the Caderneta de Saùde da Pessoa Idosa adopted the following classification:

- **Presence of a smoking risk factor**: WHO criteria were used in which **a smoker is** any individual who, at the time of the survey, has been smoking any type or quantity of tobacco on a daily basis for at least six months; and **non-smokers** are those who have never smoked, or for a short time or sporadically, any type or quantity of tobacco, at any time in their life, and are therefore not considered ex-smokers (WHO, 1992).

- **Presence of the risk factor** alcoholism: An individual who consumes more than 2 doses a day in the case of men and more than 1 dose of alcoholic drink in the case of women was considered to be an alcoholic (where 1 dose corresponds to 1 can of beer (350ml) or 1 glass of red wine (150ml) or two or more doses of distilled drink, where one dose of distilled drink corresponds to (40ml) according to the Ministry of Health (BRASIL, 2006);

- **Regular Physical Activity**: Individuals who reported doing physical activity at least three times a week for at least thirty minutes were considered to be practicing physical activity (WHO, 2003).

The Barthel index, an instrument applied through direct observation of the elderly's BADLs in the home, verified the degree of assistance required in 10 activities such as: eating, bathing, dressing, personal hygiene, defecation, urination, toilet use, chair/bed transfer, walking and stairs (O'SULLIVAN et al., 2004).

A simple overall score, ranging from 0 to 100, is calculated from the sum of all the individually weighted item scores, so that 0 is equivalent to complete dependence in all 10 activities, and 100 is equivalent to complete independence in all activities (O'SULLIVAN et al., 2004). A score of up to 20 points is categorized as "total dependence", "severe dependence" from 21 to 60 points, "moderate dependence" from 61 to 90 points, "mild dependence" from 91 to 99 points and "independence" for those who reach 100 points (SHAH et al., 1989).

This study used the Portuguese version of O'Sullivan et al. (2004), which had already been validated in Brazil. In a previous study, the instrument was subjected to reproducibility and reliability tests which showed adequate levels for the total value (MINOSSO et al., 2009).

4.6 Data collection

The team of interviewers was made up of the researcher himself, 03 students from the Geriatrics and Gerontology League of the Federal University of Maranhão, subdivided as follows: 01 student from the last period of nursing, 01 student from the fourth period of medicine and 01 student from the third period of medicine.

Training was given to the team to standardize the interviews. A pilot test was then carried out (n=10 elderly people) in order to check for any difficulties encountered by the interviewers and the elderly. After this stage, data collection began.

Data collection took place in the home environment of several neighborhoods in the city of São Luis, with elderly people enrolled in public and private sector physiotherapy programs.

After the list of addresses was made available by the Programs team, we organized the collection days, with an average of four visits per day, on Mondays, Wednesdays and Fridays.

4.7 Statistical Analysis

The data was evaluated using the statistical program *SPSS Statistics v.20* (2011).

Initially, the association between the various variables analyzed and the system, whether public or private, was evaluated using the chi-square test of independence (□^{2}). Subsequently, in order to assess the socio-demographic and lifestyle variables in the ordinal classification of the Barthel index, which measures the degree of dependence of the elderly, the Mann-Whitney and Kruskal-Wallis non-parametric tests were applied, followed by the Student-Newman-Keuls *post hoc* test for 2 x 2 comparisons.

The Mann-Whitney test was applied to assess the effect of gender, whether you live alone, whether you need care, whether you smoke, whether you drink and whether you do regular physical activity.

The Kruskal Wallis test was applied to evaluate the effect of age group, color, marital status, monthly income, who you live with, economic situation, number of people, schooling and time since joining the program. If there was a significant difference, the Student-Nenwman-Keuls *post hoc* test was applied.

Then, in order to assess the association between socio-demographic and lifestyle variables and dependency classification (Barthel index), the Chi-square test of independence (□^{2}) was used.

The significance level applied to all tests was 5%, i.e. it was considered significant when $p < 0.05$.

4.8 Ethical considerations

After authorization by the legal representative of the collection sites, the research was submitted to the Research Ethics Committee of the University Hospital of the Federal University of Maranhão (CEPHU/UFMA), and was approved under opinion number 492.583 (ANNEX C).

After clarifying the research, the participants signed the Informed Consent Form (ICF) in accordance with the requirements of Resolution 466/12 (APPENDIX A).

5 RESULTS

This systematic sample included 241 elderly people from two physiotherapy programs in the city of São Luis, 141 from the public sector and 100 from the private sector.

The time taken to admit the elderly to the physiotherapy programs in the public and private sectors varied between six months and/or more than 36 months, with 48.9% in the public sector having been there for more than 36 months and 56.0% in the private sector for less than 12 months.

Gender classification revealed a predominance of females in the two groups surveyed, with an average of 70.4%. Age ranged from 60 to 106 years, with an average of 81.7 years (SD=9.0) for the public sector and 82.5 years (SD=9.8) for the private sector. An average of 40.6% of the elderly were in the 80-89 age group. Brown was the most frequently reported color, corresponding to an average of 50.7% in the groups studied (Table 1).

Table 1 - Association of demographic variables of 241 elderly people in physiotherapy programs in the public and private sectors in Sâo Luis, Maranhâo, 2014.

Variable (n=241)	Sector Public n	%	Private n	%	p
Sex					0.065
Female	107	75,9	65	65,0	
Male	34	24,1	35	35,0	
Total	141	100,0	100	100,0	
Age					0.280
60 - 69	14	9,9	12	12,0	
70 - 79	44	31,2	20	20,0	
80 -89	54	38,3	43	43,0	
90 or more	29	20,6	25	25,0	
Total	141	100,0	100	100,0	
Age in years (Mean ± SD)	81.7 years	SD: ± 9.0	82.5 years	SD: ± 9.8	
Skin color					0.831
Brown	71	50,4	51	51,0	
White	44	31,2	33	33,0	
Black	25	17,7	16	16,0	
Yellow	1	0,7	-	-	
Total	141	100,0	100	100,0	

No statistically significant association ($p < 0.05$) was found between the type of care sector (public or private) and the demographic variables.

The data on marital status (Table 2) showed that 55.0% of the elderly in the private sector and 42.6% in the public sector were widowed (p=0.000), with 31.2% being single in the public sector. The highest incidence of elderly people with low levels of schooling (up to four years of study) was 35.5% in the public sector, while in the private sector the majority (37.0%) had over eight years or more of study, with a statistically significant difference (p=0.000).

As for the economic activities of the two groups investigated, there was a greater predominance of retired elderly people in both sectors (average of 84.5%) and no significant association was found in this variable. The monthly income of the interviewees showed a statistically significant difference (p=0.000), since in the public sector the majority (75.9%) earn one minimum wage and in the private sector the majority (43.0%) earn five or more minimum wages (Table 2).

Table 2 - Association between the social variables of the 241 elderly people in physiotherapy programs in the public and private sectors in São Luis, Maranhâo, 2014.

	Sector				
Variable (n=241)	**Public**		**Private**		**p**
	n	%	n	%	
Marital status					0.000
Viùvo	60	42,6	55	55,0	
Single	44	31,2	5	5,0	
Married	35	24,8	34	34,0	
Separate	2	1,4	6	6,0	
Total	141	100,0	100	100,0	
Education					0.000
Illiterate	43	30,5	6	6,0	
up to 4 years	50	35,5	25	25,0	
4 to 8 years	37	26.2	31	31,0	
8 or more years	11	7,8	38	38,0	
Total	141	100,0	100	100,0	
Employability					
Retired	113	80,1	89	89,0	0.125
Pensioner	19	13,5	11	11,0	
Employee	3	2,1	0	0,0	
Unemployed	2	1,4	0	0,0	
Other*	4	2,8	0	0,0	
Total	141	100,0	100	100,0	
Monthly Income					
Up to 1 Minimum Wage (MW)**	107	75,9	9	9,0	0.000
More than 1-2	27	19,1	12	12,0	
More than 2-4	5	3,5	36	36,0	
5 or more	2	1,4	43	43,0	

Total	141	100,0	100	100,0	

*Other: Continuous Cash Benefit

**Minimum wage base in 2014 (year of data collection): R$ 724,00

The distribution of the number of people living in the same household corresponds to two to four people in both the public sector (48.9%) and the private sector (65.0%). The family arrangement showed a greater predominance of elderly people living with their families in both groups (Table 3).

The place of residence of the patients assisted in the programs under analysis reflects the scope of both programs - they are patients from 70 neighborhoods distributed equally between the central (51.4%) and peripheral (48.6%) areas of the city, with 27.1% of the neighborhoods coinciding.

The majority of the elderly reported having a companion at home for most of the day (average of 87.9%), in line with the 80.9% of the elderly in the public sector and 95% of the elderly in the private sector who reported needing daily care (Table 3). A statistically significant association ($p < 0.05$) was found between the care sector (public or private) and all these variables.

Table 3 - Distribution of variables related to the support network of the 241 elderly people in public and private sector physiotherapy programs. Sâo Luis, Maranhâo, 2014.

	Sector				
Variable (n=241)	**Public**		**Private**		**p**
	n	%	n	%	
No. of people living with the elderly person					0.004
None	13	9,2	-	-	
1 person	14	9,9	11	11,0	
2-4 people	69	48,9	65	65,0	
Over 4 people	45	31,9	24	24,0	
Total	141	100,0	100	100,0	
Family arrangement					0.001
With family members	100	70,9	95	95,0	
Alone	15	10,6	1	1,0	
With friends	1	0,7	4	4,0	
Other*	25	17,7	-	-	
Total	141	100,0	100	100,0	
Alone during the day					0.001
No	114	80,9	95	95,0	
Yes	27	19,1	5	5,0	
Total	141	100,0	100	100,0	

Needs care					0.001
Yes	114	80,9	96	96,0	
No	27	19,1	4	4,0	
Total	141	100,0	100	100,0	

*Formal caregiver

The behavioral variables reported by the elderly showed that almost 100% of the elderly in both groups did not smoke and did not drink alcohol and 90% of them did not practice regular physical activity, and no significant association was found in any of these variables between the public and private care sectors (Table 4).

Table 4 - Association between the Behavioral variables of the 241 elderly people in public and private sector physiotherapy programs. Sâo Luis, Maranhâo, 2014.

Variable (n=241)	**Sector Public**		**Private**		**p**
	n	**%**	**n**	**%**	
Smoking					0.945
No	138	97,9	98	98,0	
Yes	3	2,1	2	2,0	
Total	141	100,0	100	100,0	
Alcoholic					0.232
No	139	98,6	100	100,0	
Yes	2	1,4	-	-	
Total	141	100,0	100	100,0	
Regular Physical Activity					0.894
No	129	91,5	91	91,0	
Yes	12	8,5	9	9,0	
Total	141	100,0	100	100,0	

In both groups there was an absolute predominance of positive reports of health problems among the elderly in the public and private sectors (Table 5).

Table 5 shows the morbidities according to ICD-10, highlighting the health problems self-reported by the elderly. Considering more than one answer for each interviewee, the main morbidities reported by the elderly assisted in the programs in both sectors were related to Diseases of the Circulatory System: SAH, CVA and CAD (average of 85.7%).

Diseases of the musculoskeletal system and connective tissue (arthrosis, arthritis, osteoporosis, deformities of the fingers and toes) came second in the number of reports with an average of 65.8%.

A statistically significant association ($p < 0.05$) was found between the sector of care (Public or Private) and the following ICD-10s: Symptoms, signs and abnormal findings, Diseases of the eye and appendages, Diseases of the nervous system, Mental and behavioral disorders and neoplasms.

Table 5 - Association of health problems self-reported by 241 elderly people according to ICD-10 in public and private sector physiotherapy care programs. São Luis, Maranhão, 2014.

Variable (n=241)	Sector				p
	Public		Private		
	n	%	n	%	
Health problems					0.089
Yes	137	97,2	100	100,0	
No	4	2,8	-	-	
Total	141	100,0	100	100,0	
ICD-10					
I. Diseases of the circulatory system (SAH, stroke and CAD)	122	86,5	85	85,0	0.738
2. diseases of the musculoskeletal system and connective tissue (Arthrosis, Arthritis, Osteoporosis, Toe deformity hands and feet)	87	61,7	70	70,0	0.183
3. symptoms, signs and abnormal **findings***	73	51,8	75	75,0	0.000
4. endocrine metabolic (Diabetes Mellitus, Malnutrition and Obesity)	59	41,8	42	42,0	0.981
5. diseases of the eye and appendages (visual impairment and glaucoma)	48	34,0	64	64,0	0.000
6Mental and behavioral disorders (Depression and mood disorder)	47	33,3	47	47,0	0.032
7Diseases of the nervous system (Stroke). Parkinson's, Alzheimer's and Sleep Apnea)	34	24,1	55	55,0	0.000
8. diseases of the ear and mastoid apophysis (hearing loss and labyrinthitis)	19	13,5	64	64,0	0.175
9 Diseases of the skin and subcutaneous tissue (Decubitus ulcer)	14	9,9	16	16,0	0.312
10.Diseases of the digestive system (Constipation	16	11,3	16	16,0	0.160
11.Injuries, poisoning and other external causes (amputation)	6	4,3	3	3,0	0.623
12. Diseases of the Diseases (COPD and Asthma)	4	2,8	8	8,0	0.069
13.No complaint	4	2,8	-	-	0.089
14.Neoplasms (Cancer)	3	2,1	11	11,0	0.004
15 Diseases of the genitourinary system (Cystitis)	2	1,4	-	-	0.232
16. Infectious and parasitic diseases	1	0.7	-	-	0.399

(Leprosy) *Chapter XVIII: symptoms and abnormal findings: These include dysphagia, dizziness, headache, lower back pain, cough, hair loss, aphasia.

SAH: Systemic Arterial Hypertension; CVA: Cerebrovascular Accident; CAD: Coronary Artery Disease; COPD: Chronic Obstructive Pulmonary Disease.

Table 6 shows reports of previous hospitalizations in the last 12 months among the elderly in both services, with 67% in the private sector and only 32.6% in the public sector. There were references to falls in the last 12 months among 44% of the elderly in the public sector and 25% in the private sector.

100% of the elderly in the private sector reported taking some kind of medication, and 70% reported taking five or more medications. It is noteworthy that 14.2% of the elderly in the public sector do not take any type of medication (Table 6).

These variables show a statistically significant difference ($p < 0.05$) between the care sector (Public or Private).

Table 6 - Association between reports of previous hospitalization, falls and medication consumption among the 241 elderly people monitored in public and private sector physiotherapy programs. Sâo Luis, Maranhâo, 2014.

	Sector				
Variable (n=241)	**Public**		**Private**		**p**
	n	**%**	**n**	**%**	
Prior hospitalization					0.000
No	95	67,4	33	33,0	
Yes	46	32,6	67	67,0	
Total	141	100,0	100	100,0	
Falls					0.004
No	79	56,0	75	75,0	
Yes	62	44,0	25	25,0	
Total	141	100,0	100	100,0	
Medicines					0.000
None	20	14,2	-	-	
1 - 2	28	19,9	7	7,0	
3 - 4	47	33,3	23	23,0	
5 or more	46	32,6	70	70,0	
Total	141	100,0	100	100,0	

In the private sector, around 92% of the elderly had some degree of functional dependence and in the public sector 87.9%. There was a significant association ($p < 0.05$) with the type of care sector (public or private) and the variables related to the Basic Activities of Daily Living analyzed using the Barthel index (BI). It was found that in all activities, the "dependent" classification was always higher in the private care sector (Table 7).

A significant association was found ($p < 0.05$) in the general classification of the degree of dependence (p = 0.007), assessed by the BI, showing that in the private care sector the majority (57%) have total dependence to perform BADLs, while in the public care sector only 36.9% have this degree of dependence (Table 7).

Table 7 - Association of variables related to BADL using the Barthel index in the 241 elderly people followed up in public and private sector physiotherapy programs. Sâo Luis, Maranhâo, 2014.

Barthel index (n=241)	Sector Public N	 %	 Private n	 %	 p
Food					0.000
Dependent	46	32,6	58	58,0	
Help	45	31,9	28	28,0	
Independent	50	35,5	14	14,0	
Total	141	100,0	100	100,0	
Bath					0.000
Dependent	89	63,1	88	88,0	
Help	51	36,2	12	12,0	
Independent	1	0,7	0	-	
Total	141	100,0	100	100,0	
Personal hygiene					0.000
Dependent	64	45,4	70	70,0	
Help	74	52,5	30	30,0	
Independent	3	2,1	0	-	
Total	141	100,0	100	100,0	
Clothing				0.000	
Dependent	53	37,6	69	69,0	
Help	50	35,5	22	22,0	
Independent	38	27,0	9	9,0	
Total	141	100,0	100	100,0	
Intestine				0.002	
Incontinent	48	34,0	51	51,0	
Occasional incontinence	36	25,5	29	29,0	
Continent	57	40,4	20	20,0	
Total	141	100,0	100	100,0	
Urinary Bladder				0.013	
Incontinent	52	36,9	51	51,0	
Occasional incontinence	33	23,4	27	27,0	
Continent	56	39,7	22	22,0	
Total	141	100,0	100	100,0	

("continue")

Table 7. Association of variables related to BADLs and general classification of the degree of dependence using the Barthel index in the 241 elderly people followed up in physiotherapy care programs in the public and private sectors. Sâo Luis, Maranhâo, 2014

("continuation")

Barthel index (n=241)	Sector Public n	 %	 Private n	 %	 P

Bathroom transfer					0.005
Dependent	59	41,8	63	63,0	
Great help	39	27,7	24	24,0	
Minimal help	41	29,1	13	13,0	
Independent	2	1,4	0	-	
Total	141	100,0	100	100,0	
Chair/bed transfer					0.001
Dependent	46	32,6	57	57,0	
Great help	37	26,2	20	20,0	
Minimal help	30	21,3	17	17,0	
Independent	28	19,9	6	6,0	
Total	141	100,0	100	100,0	
Mobility					0.001
Dependent	71	50,4	71	71,0	
Independent in wheelchairs	9	6,4	1	1,0	
Help	34	24,1	22	22,0	
Independent	27	19,1	6	6,0	
Total	141	100,0	100	100,0	
Stairs					
Dependent	84	59,6	76	76,0	
Help	38	27,0	19	19	,00.017
Independent	19	13,5	5	5,0	
Total	141	100,0	100	100,0	
Classification General degree of dependency				0 007	
- Independence	17	12,1	8	8,0	
- Mild dependence	11	7,8	1	1,0	
- Moderate dependence	27	19,1	11	11,0	
- Severe dependence	34	24,1	23	23,0	
- Total Dependence	52	36,9	57	57,0	
Total	141	100,0	100	100,0	

When analyzing the relationship between the degree of dependence assessed by the Barthel index and the other variables studied, considering the sector of care, a significant association ($p < 0.05$) was observed in the public sector for the following variables: alone during the day ($p = 0.001$), needs care ($p = 0.000$), drinker ($p = 0.025$), previous hospitalization ($p = 0.001$) and falls ($p = 0.015$).025), regular physical activity ($p=0.000$), previous hospitalization ($p=0.001$) and falls ($p=0.014$), while in the private sector, the variables with a statistically significant difference ($p<0.05$) were: needs care ($p=0.001$), regular physical activity ($p<0.001$) and falls ($p<0.001$) according to table 8.

Table 8 - Mann-Whitney test with the Barthel Index associated with sociodemographic and behavioral variables, previous hospitalization and occurrences of falls among 241 elderly people followed up in public and private sector physiotherapy programs. São Luis, Maranhão, 2014.

Variable (n=241)	**Public**			**Private**		
	n	**Median**	**p**	**n**	**Median**	**P**

Sex						
Male	34	Moderate/severe	0.052	35	Total Dep.	0.747
Female	107	Severa Dep.		65	Total Dep.	
Total	141			100		
Alone during the day						
No	114	Severa Dep.	n nn1	95	Total Dep.	0.314
Yes	27	Moderate Dep.	**0.00 1**	5	Severe dep.	
Total	141			100		
Needs care						
No	27	Light Dept.	**0.000**	4	Independence	**0.001**
Yes	114	Severa Dep.		96	Total Dep.	
Total	141			100		
Smoking						
No	138	Severa Dep.		98	Total Dep.	0.137
Yes	3	Moderate Dep.	0.075	2	Dep. Moderate/ Severe	
Total	141			100		
Alcoholic						
No	139	Severa Dep.		100	Total Dep.	-
Yes	2	Independence	**0.025**			
Total	141			100		
Regular physical activity						
No	129	Severa Dep.		91	Total Dep.	**< 0.001**
Yes	12	Independence/Dep. Lightweight	**0.000**	9	Light Dept.	
Total	141			100		

"continue"

Table 8 - Mann-Whitney test with the Barthel index associated with sociodemographic and behavioral variables, previous hospitalization and occurrences of falls among 241 elderly people followed up in public and private sector physiotherapy programs. Sâo Luis, Maranhâo, 2014.

("continuation")

Variable (n=241)	Public			Private		
	n	Median	p	n	Median	P
Prior hospitalization						
No	95	Moderate Dep.	0.001	33	Severa Dep.	0.175
Yes	46	Severa Dep.		67	Total Dep.	
Total	141			100		
Falls						
No	79	Severa Dep.	0.014	75	Total Dep.	< 0.001
Yes	61	Moderate Dep.		25	Severa Dep.	
Total	141			100		

Applying the Kruskall Wallis test to analyze the relationship between the degrees of dependence measured by the Barthel Index (Table 9), a significant association ($p < 0.05$) was found in the public care sector for the following variables: age (p = 0.041), marital status (p = 0.024), monthly income (p = 0.044), number of people living with the elderly person (p = 0.005).005), family arrangement (p=0.001) and medication consumption (p=0012), while in the private care sector, the variables that showed a statistically significant association (p<0.05) were: time of admission to the program (p=0.020), color (p=0.020), marital status (p=0.020) and medication consumption (0.006).

Table 9 - Kruskall Wallis test with the Barthel index associated with time of admission to the program and sociodemographic variables of the 241 elderly people monitored in public and private sector physiotherapy programs. Sâo Luis, Maranhâo, 2014.

Variable (n=241)	Public				Private			
	N	Median	SNK*	p	N	Median	SNK*	p
Time since admission to the program (months)								
≥ 6 a < 12	42	Severa Dep.			56	Severa Dep.	b	
≥ 12 a < 24	12	Total Dep.		0.485	18	Total Dep.	a	0.020
≥ 24 a < 36	18	Severa Dep.			9	Severa Dep.	b	
≥ 36	69	Severa Dep.			17	Total Dep.	a	
Total	141				100			
Age								
60 - 69	14	Moderate Dep.	b		12	Severa Dep.		
70 - 79	44	Severa Dep.	a	0.041	20	Dep. SeveraZTotal		0.391
80 - 89	54	Severa Dep.	a		43	Total Dep.		
> 89	29	Severa Dep.	a		25	Total Dep.		
Total	141				100			
Color								
Brown	71	Severa Dep.			51	Total Dep.	a	
White	44	Severa Dep.		0.347	33	Severa Dep.	b	0.020
Black	25	Severa Dep.			16	Total Dep.	a	
Yellow	1	Severa Dep.			-			
Total	141				100			
Marital status								
Viùvo	60	Severe/Total Dept.	a		55	Total Dep.	a	
Single	44	Dep. ModeradaZSevera	c		5	Total Dep.	a	
Married	35	Severa Dep.	b	0.024	34	Total Dep.	a	0.020
Separate	2	Dep. ModeradaZSevera	c		6	Severa Dep.	b	
Total	141				100			
Education								
Illiterate	43	Severa Dep.			6	Total Dep.		
up to 4 years	50	Severa Dep.		0.135	25	Severa Dep.		0.067
4 to 8 years	37	Severa Dep.			31	Total Dep.		
8 or more years	11	Moderate Dep.			37	Total Dep.		
Total	141				100			
Employability**	113	Severa Dep.		89		Total Dep.		
Retired								
Pensioner	19	Total Dep.		11		Total Dep.		
				0.443		0.546		
Employee	3	Severa Dep.		-				
Unemployed	2	Light/Moderate Dept.		-				
Other	4	Light/Moderate Dept.		-				
Total	141			100				

* SNK = Student-Newman-Keuls test.

** As there were only two classes, the Mann-Whitney test was applied to the economic situation of the private group.

"continue"

Table 9 - Kruskall Wallis test with the Barthel index associated with time of admission to the program and sociodemographic variables of the 241 elderly people monitored in public and private sector physiotherapy programs. Sâo Luis, Maranhâo, 2014.

"continuation"

Variable (n=241)	Public N	Median	SNK*	p	Private N	Median	SNK*	p
Monthly income								
Up to 1 MW	107	Severa Dep.	b		9	Severa Dep.		
More 1-2	27	Total Dep.	a	0.044	12	Dep. Severe/Total		0.365
More than 2-4	5	Severa Dep.	b		36	Total Dep.		
5 or more	2	Dep. Severe/Moderate	c		43	Total Dep.		
Total	141				100			
No. of people living with the elderly person								
None	13	Light Dept.	b		-			
1 person	14	Severa Dep.	a	0.005	11	Total Dep.		
2 - 4 people	69	Severa Dep.	a		65	Total Dep.		0.343
Over 4 people	45	Severa Dep.	a		24	Severa Dep.		
Total	141				100			
Family arrangement								
Alone	15	Moderate Dep.	b		-			
With family members	100	Severa Dep.	a	< 0.0001	95	Total Dep.		
With friends	1	Moderate Dep.	b		1	Total Dep.		0.417
Others	25	Moderate Dep.	b		4	Severa Dep.		
Total	141				100			
Medicines								
None	20	Moderate Dep.	b		-			
1 - 2	28	Severa Dep.	a	0.012	7	Moderate dep.	b	0.006
3 - 4	47	Severa Dep.	a		23	Total Dep.	a	
5 or more	46	Severa Dep.	a		70	Total Dep.	a	
Total	141				100			

* SNK = Student-Newman-Keuls test

According to the statistical analysis, among the elderly in the public sector there was a significant association (p < 0.05) with the occurrence of falls (p = 0.0391), consumption of medication (p = 0.0192) and previous hospitalization (p = 0.0008) with the degrees of severe/total dependence measured by the Barthel index (Table 10).

Table 10 - Association of the degree of dependence using the Barthel index with the occurrence of falls, consumption of medication and previous hospitalization of the 241 elderly people in the public sector physiotherapy program. Sâo Luis, Maranhâo, 2014.

Variable (n=241)	Barthel index classification Independence	%	Mild/moderate dependence	%	Severe/total dependence	%	Total	P
Falls								
No	9	11.4	15	19.0	55	69.6	79	
Yes	8	12.9	23	37.1	31	50.0	62	0,0391
Total	17		38		86		141	
Medicines								
None	7	35.0	7	35.0	6	30.0	20	
1 - 2	3	10.7	8	28.6	17	60.7	28	
3 - 4	3	6.4	11	23.4	33	70.2	47	0,0192
5 or more	4	8.7	12	26.1	30	65.2	46	

Total	17		38		86		141	
Prior hospitalization								
No	16	16.9	31	32.6	48	50.5	95	
Yes	1	2.2	7	15.2	38	82.6	46	0,0008
Total	17		38		86		141	

The elderly in the private care sector showed a significant association ($p < 0.05$) between the occurrence of falls ($p = 0.0391$) and the consumption of medication ($p = 0.0192$) and the degree of severe/total dependence measured by the Barthel index (Table 11).

Table 11 - Association of the degree of dependence using the Barthel index with the occurrence of falls, consumption of medication and previous hospitalization of the 241 elderly people in the private sector physiotherapy program. Sâo Luis, Maranhâo, 2014.

Variable (n=241)	**Barthel index classification**						**Total**	**p**
	Independence	**%**	**Mild/moderate dependence**	***D*** **o**	**Dependency severe/total**	**%**		
Falls								0,0008
No	5	6,7	5	6,7	65	86,6	75	
Yes	3	12,0	7	28,0	15	60,0	25	
Total	8		12		80		100	
Medicines								0,0052
1- 2	2	28,6	3	42,8	2	28,6	7	
3 -4	3	13,0	3	13,0	17	74,0	23	
5 or more	3	4,3	6	8,6	61	87,1	70	
Total	8		12		80		100	
Prior hospitalization								0,4109
No	4	12,1	5	15,1	24	72,8	33	
Yes	4	6,0	7	10,4	56	83,6	67	
Total	8		12		80		100	

6 DISCUSSION

This study focuses on assessing the degree of functional dependence for performing BADLs, using the Barthel index, of elderly people registered in physiotherapy programs in the public and private sectors, showing a high percentage of elderly people in both services with some degree of dependence (group average of 89.9%).

In a similar study carried out in the municipality of Guatambu (SC), the prevalence of some type of dependency was 30.5% (SANTOS et al 2007) and in a cross-sectional study of elderly members of a health plan in Rio Grande do Sul (CARDOSO; COSTA, 2010), 13.8% of the elderly had some degree of dependency. FELICIANO, MORAES and FREITAS (2004) showed a higher percentage in a prevalence study of low-income elderly people carried out in the municipality of Sâo Carlos in São Paulo (76.4% of the elderly had some degree of functional disability).

Calero et al (2011) carried out a study with 220 people living in sheltered housing for the elderly in southern Spain, obtaining an average age of 80.75 years in the interviewees, observing greater functional impairment in this age group with this average age, similarly to this study which found an average of 82.1 years in the groups surveyed, but with a greater predominance in the 80-89 age group for the elderly in the private sector (43%), which could mean that with advancing age the likelihood of the elderly presenting a greater degree of functional dependence may increase.

The differences observed between the studies can be explained by the greater or lesser access to physiotherapy services in the different Brazilian municipalities, whether offered by the public sector or by health insurance plans.

On January 4, 1994, the National Policy for the Elderly (PNI) was created with the aim of ensuring the social rights of the elderly, creating conditions to promote their autonomy, integration and effective participation in society, reaffirming their right to health at the various levels of care (SANTOS et al., 2008). One of the PNI's priorities is to encourage home care, valuing the favorable effect of the family environment on the recovery process of the elderly and providing benefits for them and the health system (SOUZA; CALDAS, 2008).

Later, other programs, such as the PNSPI, reinforced this home-based care (BRASIL, 2010). Home physiotherapy is a practice that is growing rapidly in many countries, including Brazil. There are various reasons why patients or their families opt for home physiotherapy instead of conventional care in a physiotherapy clinic, ranging from physical and functional incapacity, such as bed rest, to the convenience and practicality of this type of care (SILVA; DURAES; AZOUBEL, 2011).

Physiotherapy seeks to recover degrees of disability, promoting improvements in motor, sensory and neurological functions, offering patients greater dignity and rescuing their health (COSTA; PINHO; FIGUEIRAS; OLIVEIRA, 2009).

Studies have shown that, as the population has aged, the proportion of elderly people with sequelae of chronic degenerative diseases has also progressively increased, which generally contributes to their dependence when it comes to performing BADLs, so home care is becoming more necessary every day (BARCELO; MADUREIRA, 2009).

The results of the study carried out by Vieira et al (2013) report that the Geriatric Physiotherapy program is capable of promoting health and improving the quality of life of the elderly people it assists. These findings emphasize the importance of physiotherapy in preventing and maintaining ADLs, as well as improving quality of life. After entering the geriatric physiotherapy program, a significant proportion of the elderly experienced an improvement in their vital functions, began to exercise regularly and reduced their use of medication, which had a direct impact on their self-esteem and quality of life.

The Home Care Service at the Hospital do Servidor Pùblico municipal de Sâo

Paulo began operating in 1994. Leme and Dias (2007) pointed out the importance of home care as an alternative to the high cost of hospital admissions and the impact that the elderly population has on costs resulting from these admissions.

Although data from the PNAD shows that the functional capacity of the elderly is strongly influenced by *per capita* household income - showing that there is a relationship between worse socioeconomic status and greater inability to perform activities due to health problems (LIMA- COSTA et al, 2011), it was observed that the elderly in the public sector showed less impairment in the degree of dependence with low income and the elderly in the private sector have a higher occurrence of dependence, especially severe and total, but with higher per capita income.

There was a higher prevalence of total dependence for performing BADLs among the elderly in the private sector compared to the public sector. This can be explained by the shorter admission time of the elderly in the private sector to the physiotherapy program, with a shorter follow-up time. Although the elderly in both groups were distributed in similar age groups, the group assisted in the private sector, with a higher degree of dependence, showed a later intervention.

Like the present study, various studies have shown a predominance of women among the elderly (COSTA; NAKATANI; BACHION, 2006; SOUZA; MORAIS; BARTH, 2006; MASTROENI; ERZINGER; MASTROENI; MARUCCI, 2007). Higher male mortality, combined with female longevity, leads to a greater number of women in the elderly population. In 2010, 55.5% of the 21 million elderly were female (CAMARANO, 2011).

With regard to lifestyle habits, there was a high prevalence of not practicing regular physical activity in both groups. This confirms the large proportion of elderly people who lead sedentary lives in the country, for whom greater adherence to physical activity programs should be provided (WHO, 2005).

One of the main ways of avoiding, minimizing and/or reversing most of the physical, social and psychological declines that often accompany the elderly is physical activity, which has been shown to be constantly associated with significant improvements in health conditions, such as controlling stress, obesity, diabetes, coronary heart disease and, above all, improving the functional aptitude of the elderly (BOCALINI et al, 2008; SANTOS et al, 2007).

The elderly population in both services had a high proportion of NCDs, especially diseases of the circulatory system, with SAH and stroke being the most frequently reported. In line with the findings of this study, diseases of the circulatory system also appear as the leading cause of morbidity in the study by Monteiro et al (2013), with a percentage of 58.62 % of elderly people who attended outpatient appointments in the municipal network of Belém - PA.

According to the Sintese de Indicadores Sociais 2010, among the diseases of the circulatory system that affect the elderly, hypertension is the most frequently reported in all subgroups, with 53.3%, and is the leading cause of death in the country (IBGE, 2010a).

The high incidence of hypertension among the sample in this study is similar to that of a population study carried out by Rodrigues et al. in 2008, which found that 72.3% had SAH.

The presence of CNCDs, due to their evolutionary course, has a significant impact on both individual and collective health in the population, as well as being a determining factor in altering the functional capacity of the elderly (TAVARES; DRUMOND; PEREIRA, 2008; PEDROSA; HOLANDA, 2009).

In this way, the elderly admitted to the physiotherapy care programs in this study meet the criteria for receiving constant home care in an interdisciplinary way, as they already have some CNCD that worsens the degree of functional dependence if there is no continuity in their treatment.

Polypharmacy is a common clinical practice among the elderly. The occurrence of polypharmacy can be explained by the number of chronic diseases that affect the elderly, the high incidence of symptoms and the need for consultations and treatment with different specialists (BRASIL, 2007). Adverse drug events can compromise the functional capacity of elderly people exposed to polypharmacy, as well as representing an excess cost for the health system (ROZENFELD; FONSECA; ACURCIO, 2008).

Carvalho et al (2012) report that medicines can help maintain functional capacity, but they can also compromise it. For this reason, the drugs to be prescribed for the elderly should have their benefit-risk ratio well assessed.

This study shows that most of the elderly in the private sector take polypharmacy, possibly due to greater access to medical care at home and the ease with which they can seek treatment from various specialists. In the private sector, 14.2% do not consume any type of medication, due to the fact that the program team includes a geriatrician who accompanies the elderly at home and assesses the appropriate medication, thus avoiding polypharmacy.

The Interdisciplinary Home Care Center (NADI) at the Hospital das Clinicas of the Faculty of Medicine of the University of São Paulo is staffed by geriatricians and those trained in palliative care. Resident doctors from medicine and geriatrics also take part in home care and, under the guidance of the assistant, coordinate medical visits. The target group is mostly frail elderly people (MANGUEIRA, 2010).

Care is provided through clinical, socioeconomic and cognitive questioning, as well as a physical examination, assessment of the patient's current functionality, a list of medications and verification of the environment and family relationships. Interdisciplinarity brings the benefit of humanizing care and is the most important aspect of medical care at NADI (MANGUEIRA, 2010).

The inclusion of the geriatrician with the interdisciplinary team in home care programs for the elderly in public and private sector care services is of great importance for the development of treatment for the elderly who have lost some degree of functional dependence.

In this study, there was a high number of hospital admissions among the elderly in the private sector when compared to the elderly in the public sector over the last twelve months. There is evidence of the frequent involvement of hospitalizations in worsening the functional condition of the elderly (GIACOMIN et al, 2010). This may be another factor related to a higher degree of functional dependence.

With regard to the occurrence of falls in the last 12 months, the elderly in the public sector had a higher proportion of this event than the elderly in the private sector in the same period. Padoin et al (2010) report a rate of falls among the elderly of around 30% per year, which may increase with advancing age.

The occurrence of falls is one of the main disabling factors in the elderly, causing restrictions in activities of daily living according to studies carried out by Ribeiro et al (2008), Beck et al (2011) and Ganança (2006). A group of elderly people in the public sector remain alone during the day (around 20%), which may be related to the higher number of falls observed among elderly people in this sector.

Studying the clinical and functional profile of the elderly in a physiotherapeutic care program, paying attention to the differences that exist between the groups cared for in the public and private sectors, is essential, since preventive strategies can be adopted to address the specific needs of this population, so that they can prolong their lives with quality, minimizing the degree of functional incapacity.

In the field of physiotherapy, the focus of care for the elderly in physiotherapy programs needs to be broadened. Certainly, physiotherapy interventions will be more effective as its field of action becomes more comprehensive and specific.

This study had limitations with regard to the collection of self-reported morbidities by the elderly in the public and private sectors in physiotherapy care programs, which may underestimate the prevalence of morbidities due to cognitive problems or even lack of diagnosis, which was sometimes reported by the elderly person's guardian.

7 CONCLUSION

The study showed that the elderly in both services are experiencing aging characterized by: a high prevalence of chronic non-communicable diseases, evolving with functional loss and a predominance of females.

There was a greater degree of dependence when it came to performing Basic Activities of Daily Living among the elderly in the private sector compared to the public sector, which could be explained by the shorter time that the elderly in the private sector were admitted to the physiotherapy program and the shorter follow-up time.

This demonstrates the importance of prolonging and improving the quality of life of the elderly by expanding home-based programs with interdisciplinary assistance for this age group.

REFERENCES

ALVES, L. C. et al. The influence of chronic diseases on the functional capacity of the elderly in the municipality of Sâo Paulo, Brazil. **Cad Saùde Pùblica**, v.23, n.8, p. 1924-1930, aug., 2007.

ARALDI, Marilani. **Discovering life projects** - the contribution of the elderly entrepreneur project to the ageing process. Social Work Course Conclusion Paper, UFSC. Florianópolis: 2008.

ARAUJO LF et al. Evidence of the contribution of elderly support programs to healthy aging in Brazil. **Rev Panam Salud Publica**, v.30, n.1, p.80-86, 2011.

ARAÙJO, K. B. G. **The rescue of memory in work with the elderly:** the role of physical education. Master's dissertation. Campinas: Faculty of Physical Education, UNICAMP, 2001.

WORLD BANK (IBRD) - International Bank for Reconstruction and Development (Brazil Department). **Ageing in an Older Brazil**. Implications of Population Ageing on: Economic Growth, Poverty Reduction, Public Finances, Service Delivery. 2011.

BARCELOS, E.M.; MADUREIRA, M.D.S. Sindrome da Imobilidade, p.153160. In-CHAIMOWICZ, F.et al. **Saùde do Idoso: Envelhecimento Populacional e Saùde dos Idosos**. 1.ed.Belo Horizonte: Coopmed, 2009, 172p.

BARROS, M. B. A. et al. Social inequalities in the prevalence of chronic diseases in Brazil, PNAD-2003. **Cienc Saùde Coletiva**, v.11, n.4, p. 911926, oct./dec., 2006.

BEAUVOIR, Simone de. **Old Age**: an uncomfortable reality. Sâo Paulo: Difusâo Européia, Volume, 1970.

BRAZIL. Ministry of Health. Ordinance No. 73 of May 10, 2001. Norms for the operation of elderly care services in Brazil. **Official Gazette of the Union**, Brasilia, May 14, 2001. Section 1.

BRAZIL. Ministry of Health. **Caderneta de saùde da pessoa Idosa**. Brasilia: Ministry of Health; 2012.

BRAZIL. Ministry of Health. **Caderneta de saùde da pessoa Idosa**. Brasilia: Ministry of Health; 2007.

BRAZIL. Ministry of Health. **Statute of the elderly**. Paulo Paim (org). Brasilia: Federal Senate. Undersecretariat for Technical Publications, 2003. 68 p.

BRAZIL. Ministry of Health. Secretariat of Health Care, Department of Primary Care. Cadernos da Atençâo Bàsica, n.19. **Ageing and health of the elderly**. Brasilia: Ministry of Health. 2010.

CARVALHO FILHO, E.T.; PAPALEO NETTO, M. **Geriatria:** fundamentos, clinica e terapèutica. Sâo Paulo: Atheneu, 2000.

CARLETO, D. G. S. et al. Estrutura da pràtica da terapia ocupacional: dominio e processo - 2ª edição. **Revista Triângulo**, Uberaba, v. 3, n. 2, p. 57-147, 2010.

ICD10. International Code of Diseases - Tenth Revision - 2000. **ICD 10**. Available at: http://www.datasus.gov.br/cid10/webhelp/cid10.htm. Accessed on: September 30, 2014. 2014.

FERNANDES, H.C. **Access to health services and its relationship with functional capacity and frailty in elderly people assisted by the Family Health Strategy.** Dissertation (Master of Science). Sâo Paulo: University of Sâo Paulo, 2010

FHON, J.R.S.; WEHBE, S.C.C.F.; VENDRUSCOLO, T.R.P.; STACKFLETH

R.; MARQUES S.; RODRIGUES, R.A.P. Falls in the elderly and their relationship with functional capacity. **Rev. Latino-Am. Enfermagem**, v.20, n.5, Sept./Oct. 2012.

FHON. J.R.S.; DINIZ, M.A.; LEONARDO, K.C.; KUSUMOTA, L.; HAAS, VJ.; RODRIGUES, R.A.P. Sindrome de fragilidade relacionada à incapacidade funcional no idoso. **Acta Paul Enferm**. 2012; 00 (0)

FIEDLER, M.M.; PERES, K.G. Functional capacity and associated factors in elderly people in southern Brazil: a population-based study. **Caderno de Saùde Pùblica**, Rio de Janeiro, v.24, n.2, p.409-415, feb. 2008.

FONSECA, JEC. The elderly and medicines. **Saùde em Revista** (UNIMEP), v. 2, n.4, p.35-41, 2000.

FREESE, E. M.; FONTBONNE, A. Comparative epidemiological transition: vulnerability, precariousness and Vulnerability. In: FREESE, E. M. **Epidemiologia, politicas e determinates das doenças crônicas não transmissiveis no Brasil**. Recife: Ed. Universitària da UFPE, 2006. chap. 1.

FREITAS, F.; COSTA, S.H.M.; RAMOS, J.G.L.; MAGALHAES, J.A. **Rotinas em obstetricia**. 6th ed. Porto Alegre: Artmed, 2011.

FREITAS, E.V.; PY, L.; CANÇADO, F.A.X.; DOLL, J.; GORZONI, M.L. **Tratado de Geriatria e Gerontologia**. 2.ed. Rio de Janeiro: Guanabara Koogan, 2006. 1666p.

FREITAS, E.V.; MIRANDA, R.D. Comprehensive Geriatric Assessment. IN: FREITAS et al. **Tratado de Geriatria e Gerontologia**. Rio de Janeiro: Guanabara Koogan, 2011.

GOMES, S.de.S. **Dificuldades vivenciadas por cuidadores informais** de **idosos dependentes assistidos pelo Serviço de Assistência Domiciliar (SAD/SUS) do Hospital Cardoso Fontes, no município do Rio de Janeiro/Rj.** Dissertation (Master's in Family Health) - Estàcio de Sá University, Rio de Janeiro, 2012. 99p.

GONTIJO, S. **Envelhecimento ativo:** uma política de saù/World Health Organization; Brasilia: Organizaçâo Pan-Americana da Saù, 2005.

BRAZILIAN INSTITUTE OF GEOGRAPHY AND STATISTICS. **In 30 years, the NE has the greatest gain in life expectancy: 12.95 years**. Rio de Janeiro, 2013. Available at:

<http://saladeimprensa.ibge.gov.br/noticias?view=noticia&id=1&idnoticia=2436. Accessed on: May 4, 2014.

. **2010 demographic census**: results of the population characteristics sample. Available at: http://www.cidades.ibge.gov.br. Accessed on: May 22, 2014.

. **Synthesis of social indicators**: an analysis of the living conditions of the Brazilian population 2010. Available at: http://www.ibge.gov.br/home/estatistica/populaca/condicaodevida/indicadoresminimos/sinteseindicsocial2010/SIS-2010.pdf. Accessed on: April 20, 2014.

KALACHE AND KICKBUSCHH. **Active Ageing**: a policy framework, 1997.

KARSCH, UMS. Dependent elderly: families and caregivers. **Cadernos de Saùblica** 2003; 19(3): 861-866.

KAWASAKI, K.; DIOGO, M.J.D. The use of the Functional Independence Measure (FIM) in the elderly: a literature review. **Med Reabil**, 2004: 23(3):57-60.

LEME, L.E.G.; DIAS, M.H.M.da.S. Home Care Service: objectives, organization and results. In: PAPALÉO NETTO, M. **Tratado de gerontologia.** 2nd ed. Sâo Paulo: Atheneu, 2007. Chap.54. p.683-694

LITVOC, J; BRITO, FC. Functional capacity. In: LITVOC, J; BRITO, FC. **Ageing**: prevention and health promotion. Sâo Paulo: Atheneu, 2004. P.17-35.

MACIEL ACC, GUERRA, RO. Influence of biopsychosocial factors on the functional capacity of elderly residents in northeastern Brazil. **R. Bras. Epidemiol.**, v.10, p.179-89, 2007.

MARQUES, B. **Quem ama se cuidida**: Life and health. Santa Maria: Franciscan University Center, 2001.

MAZO, G.Z.; LOPES, M.A.; BENEDETTI, T.B. **Atividade fisica e o idoso:** concepçâo gerontològica. Porto Alegre: Sulina, 2001.

MC DOWEL I.; NEWELL, C. **Measuring health:** a guide to rating scales and questionaires. 2nd ed. New York: Oxford University Press; 1996.

MENDES, E. V. **As redes de atençâo à saù**. 2a. ed. Brasilia: Pan American Health Organization, 2011.

MINISTRY OF HEALTH. **Ordinance No. 2.528 of October 19, 2006.**

Approves the National Health Policy for the Elderly. Brasilia: MS; 2006.

Available at:

http://www.saudeidoso.icict.fiocruz.br/pdf/PoliticaNacionaldeSaudedaPessoaI dosa.pdf. Accessed on: February 10, 2015.

MINOSSO, J.S.M.; AMENDOLA, F.; ALVARENGA, M.R.M.; OLIVEIRA, M.A. de.C. Prevalence of functional incapacity and dependence in elderly people treated at a health center-school of the University of Sâo Paulo.

Cogitare Enferm. Sâo Paulo. v.15, n.1, p.12-18, Jan/Mar, 2010.

. Validation of the Barthel index in elderly outpatients in Brazil. **Acta Paul Enferm**. In press 2009.

MORAES, E. **Health care for the elderly:** conceptual aspects. Brasilia: Pan American Health Organization, 2012.

MORAES, E.N. **Principios bàsicos de gerontologia e geriatria**. Belo Horizonte: Coopmed, 2008. p. 21-25.

MOTTA, L.B et al. Basic concepts on aging. Health of the Elderly, Module 1, unit 3.**UFMA/UNASUS**. Sâo Luis, 2013.

NERI, Anita Liberalesso. **Key words in gerontology**. Campinas: Alinea, 2001.

NETTO, MPB. **Emergencies in geriatrics:** epidemiology, pathophysiology, clinical picture, therapeutic management. São Paulo: Atheneu, 2001.

WORLD HEALTH ORGANIZATION. **Active ageing:** a health policy. Brasilia: Pan American Health Organization, 2005.

O'SULLIVAN, Susan B; SCHMITZ, Thomas J; LOPES, Fernando Augusto; RIBEIRO, Lilia Breternitz. **Fisioterapia:** avaliaçâo e tratamento. 2a. ed. Sâo Paulo: Manole, 2004.

PAIXÂO JÙNIOR CM, REICHENHEIM ME. A review of instruments for assessing the functional status of the elderly. **Cad Saùde Pùblica,** Rep Public Health. v.21, n.1, p.7-19, 2005.

PAPALÉO NETTO, M. Aging Process and Longevity. In: PAPALÉO NETTO, M. **Tratado de gerontologia.** 2nd ed. Sâo Paulo: Atheneu, 2007. Chapter 1.

PARKER, M.G.; THORSLUND, M. Health trends in the elderly population: getting better and getting worse. **Gerontologist.** Oxford, v. 47, n. 2, p. 150-8, 2007

PASCHOAL, S.. Autonomy and Independence. IN: PAPALÉO NETTO, M.. **Gerontology**. Sâo Paulo: Atheneu Publishing House, 2005.

PEREIRA, L.S.M.; GOMES, G.C. Functional assessment. In: CUNHA, U.G.V.; GUIMARÂES, R.M. **Sinais e sintomas em geriatria.** Sâo Paulo, Rio de Janeiro, Ribeirâo Preto, Belo Horizonte: Atheneu, 2004. Chapter 3

PERRACINI, M.R., FLÓ, C.M., GUERRA, R.O., Functionality and Ageing. In: PERRACINI, M.R., FLÓ, C.M., GUERRA, R.O., **Functionality and ageing - physiotherapy:** theory and clinical practice. Rio de Janeiro: Guanabara Koogan, 2009. Chap.1. p.3-24.

NATIONAL HOUSEHOLD SAMPLE SURVEY 2013. Available at: http://www.ibge.gov.br/home/. Accessed on: September 18, 2014.

RAMOS, L.R. Determinants of healthy aging in elderly urban residents: Epidoso Project, Sâo Paulo. **Cadernos de Saùde Pùblica**, Rio de Janeiro, v. 19, n. 3, p.793-797, jun. 2003.

RICI, N.A.; KUBOTA, M.T.; CORDEIRO, R.C. Concordance of observations on the functional capacity of elderly people in home care.

Rev.Saùde Pùblica, Sâo Paulo, Aug 2005, 39 (4).

ROLIM, F.S.; FORTI, V.A.M. Ageing and Physical Activity: helping to improve and maintain quality of life. In: DIOGO D'ÉLBOUX, M.J.; NERI, A.L.; CACHIONI, M. (Orgs). **Health and quality of life in old age.** Campinas, SP: Alinea, 2004. p.57-73

ROZENFELD S, FONSECA MJM, ACURCIO FA. Drug utilization and polypharmacy among the elderly: a survey in Rio de Janeiro City, Brazil. **Pan Am J Public Health**, v.23, p.34-43, 2008.

SALGADO, Marcelo Antonio. Groups and pedagogical action in social work with the elderly. Public policies for housing the elderly. **A Terceira Idade**, v. 39, Sâo Paulo, 2007.

SANTANA MC, CUPERTINO APFB, NERI AL. Meanings of religiosity according to community-dwelling elderly. **Geriat & Geront**., v.3, n.2, p.7077, 2009.

SANTANA, Christiane M. Aspectos Clinicos na Pràtica Geriàtrica. In: PEREIRA, Carlos U.; ANDRADE FILHO, A. de S. **Neurogeriatria**. Rio de Janeiro: Revinter, 2001. p. 46-50.

SANTOS, S.S.C.; BARLEM, E.L.D.; SILVA, B.T.; CESTARI, M.E.; LUNARDI, V.L. Promoting the health of the elderly: a commitment of gerontogeriatric nursing. **Acta Paulista de Enfermagem**, v.21, n.4, p.649-653, 2008.

SANTOS, A.M.; GAETA, P. Comprehensive Geriatric Assessment. In: FALCAO, L.F.dos.R.; COSTA, L.H.D.C.; Filho, C.de.M.A.F et al. **Manual** de **Geriatria**. Sâo Paulo: Roca, 2012. Chap. 1. p.1-10.

SHAH, S., VANCLAY, F., COOPER, B. (1989). Improving the sensitivity of the Barthel Index for stroke rehabilitation. **Journal of Clinical Epidemiology**, 42(8), 703-709.

SILVA, V. **Velhice e envelhecimento:** qualidade de vida para os idosos inseridos nos projetos do Sesc-Estreito. Florianópolis: Federal University of

Santa Catarina, 2009. 71 p. (Course Conclusion Work - Graduation in Social Work). Available at: <http://tcc. bu. ufsc. br/Ssocial287076. pdf> Accessed on Oct. 10, 2014.

SILVA, L.W.S.; DURAES. A.M.; AZOUBEL, R. Fisioterapia domiciliar: pesquisa sobre o estado da arte a partir do Niefam. **Fisioter Mov**. Curitiba, v.24, n.3, p.495-501, jul/set. 2011.

SOUZA, I.R.; CALDAS, C.P. Gerontological home care: contributions to the care of the elderly in the community. **RBPS**, v.21, n.1, p.61-68, 2008.

STIAVALI M. Supplementary health regulation and the age structure of beneficiaries. **Ciênc. Saùde Coletiva**, v.16, n.9, p.3729-3739, 2011.

STRAUB, R. H., CUTOLO, M., ZIETZ, B et al. The Process of aging chages the interplay of the immune endocrine and nervous sytem. **Mech Ageing Develop**. 2010; 122: 1591-1611.)

TEIXEIRA, Indo. **Biological Frailty and Quality of Life in Old Age**. In: Neri Al. Quality of life in old age: A multidisciplinary approach. Alinea. Campinas, 2007.

TORRES, M.V. Functional Capacity and Ageing. IN: MALAGUTTI et al. **Interdisciplinary Approach to the Elderly**. Rio de Janeiro: Rubio, 2010.

TRIBESS, S.; VIRTUOSO JUNIOR, J. S.; PETROSKI, E. L. Factors associated with physical inactivity in elderly women in low-income communities. **Rev. Salud Pùblica**, v.11, n.1. p. 39-49. Jan./Feb., 2009.

VERAS, R. Contemporary population aging: demands, challenges and innovations. **Rev. Saùde Pùblica**, v.43, n.3, p. 548-554, 2009.

VERAS, R.P, et al. New paradigms of the care model in the health sector: consequence of the population explosion of the elderly in Brazil. In: VERAS, R.(Org.) **Terceira Idade: gestao contemporànea em saù**. Rio de Janeiro: Relume-Dumarà; UNATI/UERJ, 2002. p.11-8.

VIEIRA, G.C.M. VASCONCELOS, R.dos.S.; CHAVES, R.G.; MOREIRA, M.de.F.A.da.P.; NOGUEIRA, M.M.; CÂMARA, T.M.da.S.; BASTOS, V.P.D. Geriatric physiotherapy program as a promoter of health and quality of life.**Revista Brasileira de qualidade de vida**. v. 05, n. 01, jan./jun. 2013, p. 36-43

WORLD HEALTH ORGANIZATION (WHO). Geneva; 2009. Available at: http://www.who.int/en. Accessed on October 20, 2014.

WORLD HEALTH ORGANIZATION (WHO). **Diet, nutrition and prevention of chronic diseases**. Report of a Joint WHO/FAO Expert Consultation.

Geneva: World Health Organization; 2003.

WORLD HEALTH ORGANIZATION. **Guidelines for the conduct of the tobacco smoking surveys of the general population**: report of a meeting. Geneva, 1992.

ANNEX A- HEALTH BOOKLET FOR THE ELDERLY.

Evaluation Instrument - Research Protocol.

Functionality of the Elderly at Home in a Situation of Frailty.

Questionnaire Number: _____ **Date of Interview:** / /2014.

Name :____

Address:____

Neighborhood: Zip code: ________

Phone:______________________________

Prompt:____________

Type of service: (1) Public (PADIF) (2) Private (GEAP)

Admission to the Program: // ___

( ) **≥6 months and < 12 months**

( ) **≥12 months <24 months**

( ) **≥24 months <36 months**

( ) **≥36 months**

SOCIODEMOGRAPHIC VARIABLES

1.Sex: (1) Male (2) Female

2 Date of Birth:_________/___ // **AGE:** __________________

3. COLOR: (1) White (2) Black (3) Brown (4) Yellow (5) Indigenous

4. marital status: (1) married (2) single (3) widowed (4) separated or divorced

5. schooling (E): (1) illiterate (2) up to 4 years (3) 4 to 8 years (4) 8 years or more

6.Economic Situation (ES): (1) Employed (2) Unemployed (3) Retired (4) Pensioner (5) Other

7. Monthly Income (MA): (1) Up to 1 minimum wage (MW) (2) More than 1 - 2 MW (3) More than 2 - 4 MW (4) More than 5 MW

8 Number of people living with the elderly person: (1) None (2) only 1 (3) between 2 and 4 (4) over 4

7 Do you live: (1) Alone (2) With family (3) With friends (4) Other___________________________

(Formal Caregiver)

8. Are you alone most of the day? (0) no (1) yes

9. Do you need daily care? (0) no (1) yes

BEHAVIORAL VARIABLES (lifestyle)

1.**Smoking:** (0) No (1) Yes

2. **Alcoholism**: (0) No (1) Yes	
3. **Do you practice any type of physical activity**: (0) No (1) Yes	
PERSONAL MORBIDITY DATA	
1)Existing health problem: (0) No (1) Yes **Report the presence or absence of the following health problems ?** (1) Hypertension (2) Diabetes (3) Arthrosis (4) Arthritis (5) Osteoporosis (6) Chronic Obstructive Pulmonary Disease (7) Stroke (8) Other: ________________________	
2. Quantity of medicines: (1) None (2) 1 - 2 medicines (3) 3 - 4 medicines (4) 5 or more medicines	
3. Have you been hospitalized in the last 12 months? 0) No (1) Yes	
4. Have you reported any falls in the last 12 months? (0) No (1) Yes	

ANNEX B - BARTHEL INDEX

ACTIVITY	SCORE
1)FOOD (0) DEPENDENT. (5) HELP. Need help with cutting, buttering etc. (10) INDEPENDENT Able to use any cutlery. Eats in reasonable time.	
2)BATHING (0) DEPENDENT. (5) INDEPENDENT. Wash yourself completely in the shower or bath, or use the sponge all over your body. Gets in and out of the bath. Can do everything without help from another person.	
3) PERSONAL HYGIENE (0) DEPENDENT. (5) INDEPENDENT. Wash your face, hands, brush your teeth, etc. Shave and use the socket without any problem in the case of an electrical appliance.	
4)CLOTHING (0) DEPENDENT. (5) HELP. Needs help, but completes at least half of the tasks in reasonable time. (10) INDEPENDENT. Dresses, undresses and tidies up. Ties shoe laces. Fits hernia belt or corset if necessary.	
5)INTESTINE (0) INCONTINENT (5) OCCASIONAL INCONTINENT. Has occasional episodes of incontinence or needs help using a probe or other device. (10) CONTINENT. He has no episodes of incontinence. If enemas or suppositories are needed, he puts them in by himself.	
6)URINARY BLADDER (0) INCONTINENT (5) OCCASIONAL INCONTINENT. Has occasional episodes of incontinence or needs help using a probe or other device. (10) CONTINENT. No episodes of incontinence. When he uses a tube or other device, he	

makes his own arrangements.	
7)TRANSFERS IN THE BATHROOM (0) DEPENDENT. (5) HELP. Needs help to maintain balance, clean herself and put her clothes on. (10) INDEPENDENT. Uses the toilet or urinal. Sits and stands up unaided (although uses grab rails). Cleans and dresses without help.	
8)CHAIR AND BED TRANSFERS (0) DEPENDENT. (05) GREAT HELP. Can sit up, but needs full assistance to pass. (10) MINIMAL HELP. Needs minimal help or supervision. (15) INDEPENDENT. He doesn't need any help; if he uses a wheelchair, he does so independently.	
9)MOBILITY (0) DEPENDENT. (05) INDEPENDENT IN A WHEELCHAIR. Moves around in a wheelchair for at least 50m. (10) HELP. Can walk up to 50m, but needs help or supervision. (15) INDEPENDENT. They can walk unaided for up to 50m, although they use walking sticks, crutches, prostheses or a walker.	
10)LADDERS (0) DEPENDENT. (5) HELP. Needs physical help or supervision. (10) INDEPENDENT. They are able to go up or down stairs without help or supervision, although they do need devices such as crutches or a cane or to lean on the handrail.	
Total score (PT): 100 points **(1)100 points - Independence** **(2)91 to 99 points - Mild dependence** **(3)61 to 90 points - Moderate Dependence** **(4)21 to 60 points - Severe Dependence** **(5)Less than or equal to 20 - Total Dependence**	**PT:** **Classification:**

Source: SHAH, S., VANCLAY, F., COOPER, B. (1989). Improving the sensitivity of the Barthel Index for stroke rehabilitation. **Journal of Clinical Epidemiology**, 42(8), 703-709.

APPENDICES

APPENDIX A - Informed Consent Form.

Dear Sir or Madam

You are being invited to take part in a research study on: **"Functionality of the elderly at home in situations of frailty"**, carried out by Master's student: Adriano Filipe Barreto Grangeiro, under the supervision of Prof. Mônica Elinor Alves Gama.

This research is justified by the fact that elderly people are more exposed to diseases, compromising their functional capacity and making them totally dependent on their daily activities.

The aim of this research is to study the clinical and functional profile of frail elderly people in home physiotherapy programs in the public and private sectors.

The study will be carried out as follows: after you agree to take part in the study, we will fill in the Elderly Person's Health Booklet and the Barthel index, where you will need to answer some questions about your age, sex, marital status, education, occupational situation, personal health data, lifestyle habits, falls and basic activities of daily living.

I would like to make it clear that this research is independent of your treatment and will have no influence on you if you do not agree to take part. Therefore, your participation in this study is voluntary and you will not incur any costs or reimbursements.

You will have the guarantee of receiving clarification on any questions related to the research, access to your data at any stage of the study, total freedom to refuse participation or withdraw your consent at the time of the research without any harm to the people involved in this work, as well as answering any question that you find embarrassing.

The information you provide will be kept confidential, the identity of the participants will be kept confidential, the data collected will only be used for scientific purposes in order to meet the objectives of the research, and only the general results may be published without identification in a health journal, as well as being presented at symposiums and/or congresses.

They will be published anonymously and together with the responses of the other participants. We ask for your permission to share your image in case it is necessary for proof and better explanation of the scientific work.

This study poses risks to the research subjects, possibly related to discomfort in sharing information or discomfort in talking about certain subjects. If any question makes you feel uncomfortable and you want to withdraw, you can stop taking part in the research if you wish, without any embarrassment. Risks will be minimized as the research will be ethically monitored and supervised by a qualified team.

If you agree to take part in this research, you may benefit from reflecting on this phase of your life or having a moment to share your experience and feelings related to ageing, thus prolonging your life and achieving a better quality of life with greater autonomy and independence.

It is hoped that with your participation, knowledge will be produced from the data provided, contributing to decision-making in the management of health care services for the elderly in our municipality.

If you have any questions about the research, you can contact the supervisor, Prof. Mônica Elinor Alves Gama, at any time by calling: (98) 3216-9900 and the researcher in charge, Adriano Filipe Barreto Grangeiro, by calling: (98) 3243-2912.

If you have any questions about your ethical rights and the National Health Council Resolution, please contact the Ethics Committee for Research on Human Beings of the Presidente Dutra University Hospital (CEP-HUUFMA) on (98) 2109-1250, Monday to Friday, from 8:00 a.m. to 12:00 p.m. and from 2:00

p.m. to 5:00 p.m. and speak to Prof. Dorlene Maria.

The researchers in this study undertake to comply with Resolution 466/12 on research involving human beings.

Therefore, if you agree to take part in the research as stated in the explanations and guidelines above, please put your name in the place indicated below.

We would like to thank you for your cooperation and ask you to sign and initial this form, which will also be signed and initialed by the researcher in charge in two copies, one of which will remain with you and the other with the researcher in charge.

Certificate of consent:

Name of participant: ____

Having received all the necessary information, I freely and spontaneously agree to take part in this research, and I inform you that I have signed and received a copy of this document.

Participant's signature or digital signature: ______________________

Signature or digital signature of the person responsible:

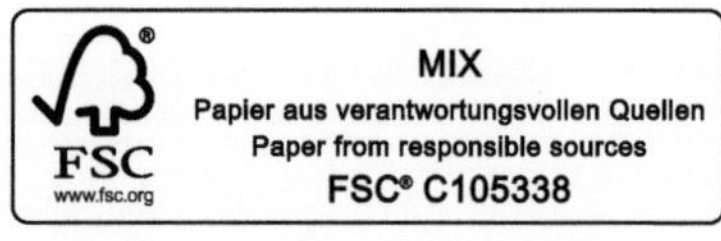

Printed by Books on Demand GmbH, Norderstedt / Germany